Someone I Love Has ALS:

A Family Caregiver Guide

Edited by Jodi O'Donnell Ames

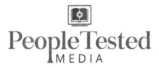

PeopleTested
MEDIA

Table of Contents

Editor's Introduction

By Jodi O'Donnell-Ames,
former caregiver, patient advocate

I had never heard of ALS or Amyotrophic Lateral Sclerosis before that last weekend in May 1995, which started the Memorial Day weekend and for many families, vacation plans. Most families were packing sunblock, fireworks, hot dogs and swimsuits and heading to the beach, but my late husband Kevin O'Donnell and I were at the hospital, demanding an answer after eight months of uncertainty. Nearly one year before, he was playing touch football with his friends and fell several times. Months later he got extremely worried when, for the first time in his life, he could not ski. When he fell on those skis, he couldn't get up. More symptoms began. Kevin could see and feel tiny muscle twitches taking place on his legs; we later learned their neurological term, fasciculations.

After seeing a primary doctor, then someone in sports medicine, we finally ended up in the office of a top neurologist who would rather tell us the news after the holiday. This journey is a common story told by many patients. I do not blame anyone for not wanting to share this news, and there is no quick diagnostic tool for ALS. First, many other possibilities must be eliminated. But after so many long doctors' appointments and leaving our toddler daughter Alina with countless friends and family members, we needed an answer. We had not heard of ALS until that day and had no idea how much those three letters would change our lives forever. I will never forget our ride home in tears.

We drove to pick up Alina from my parents' house and words like terminal, sporadic, feeding tube, and ventilator were exploding in my head. It was a surreal drive and in many ways, one that would prepare us for many similar drives. When the three of us were home, we called our loved ones and asked if we could pray together. There was no reason to ask, they were there in a heartbeat.

My late husband Kevin battled ALS for six years and was my hero. He lost his ability to walk without assistance one year after diagnosis. He depended on a wheelchair shortly after. The need for a wheelchair was followed by the placement of a feeding tube when Kevin's ability to swallow was taken. Eventually, Kevin relied on a ventilator and lost the ability to speak. Even though Kevin lost his speech, he never lost his sense of humor, and we read his lips to communicate his every need, emotions, and even jokes. We read that he loved us. We read that he was in pain. We read his lips so that he could continue his role as a Loan Analyst and employee of TD Bank (then Commerce). Kevin's job and his determination to provide for us, along with his employer's patience, had kept us insured and in our home. While most everything was stripped from the man I loved, Kevin and his love for life, remained constant. He loved the Philadelphia Eagles, Ford Mustangs, Steely Dan and his family and friends, and continued to be there for us. He welcomed parties in our home even after he could no longer enjoy a cold beer. He attended a concert even though he couldn't sing along. He played pranks at Halloween, from his wheel-chair, vent and all, he snuck out from behind a haunted garage and truly frightened trick-or-treaters before we gave them their candy.

This guide was created by a variety of caregivers and professionals who have years of experience with various aspects of ALS. It was written over many months, by volunteers who care about ALS and your journey.

It is the resource that I wish we had received along with the shocking diagnosis.

From that day in 1995 and forward, Kevin's battle was also my battle. WE battled ALS. I say we because if you live with ALS, so does your family. It takes a whole village of family and friends, big hearts and even bigger acts of courage to love and care for someone with ALS.

I tell those who are brave enough to ask me about my six years as a caregiver that I would do it again without hesitation. My role was so difficult yet so meaningful; to be Kevin's wife, friend, caregiver and advocate as well as his arms, legs, hands and voice was a humbling gift. Not a day goes by that I do not think of him and thank him for his love, courage and trust.

We share this book with you and your family with admiration and respect. Whether you are a caregiver or a patient, I hope something inside the following pages will be useful to you and your family.

"Nothing is impossible to a willing heart."
John Heywood

CHAPTER 1

What is ALS?

By Dr. Terry Heiman-Patterson, M.D.

Amyotrophic Lateral Sclerosis (more commonly referred to as Lou Gehrig's disease) is a neuromuscular disease that causes damage to the nerve cells controlling voluntary muscle movement, also known as motor neurons. It belongs to a group of diseases known as motor neuron diseases that affect the motor system. To understand ALS and the spectrum of motor neuron diseases, this book will review the motor system, what the signs and symptoms of motor system damage are, and the different motor system diseases (Table 1). This will set the stage for an in-depth discussion of ALS including the clinical picture, possible causes, and treatment of the disease.

ALS is a disease that affects the motor system, a tag team of motor nerve cells (motor neurons) that carry messages from the area that controls movement in the brain to the muscle (Figure 1). The first part of the motor system carries the signal from the brain to the lower part of the brain (brainstem) and the spinal cord. It's referred to as the upper motor neuron (UMN) or corticospinal tract. The upper motor neuron contacts a second motor neuron referred to as the lower motor neuron (LMN) or anterior horn cell. The LMN then carries the signal to the muscle. The LMNs in the brainstem contact the muscles responsible for speech and swallowing. Involvement of this area is called bulbar involvement. The highest part of the spinal cord is known as the cervical cord, and motor neurons in this area send messages to the arm muscles and diaphragm (one of the muscles important for breathing). The middle part of the spinal cord is called the thoracic cord and neurons here innervate (control) the muscles of the trunk and the muscles of the chest important for breathing. The lowest part of the spinal cord is the lumbar spinal cord and the motor nerves at this level innervate the leg muscles.

It is possible to determine that there is motor neuron damage by the symptoms that a person has along with the examination of the motor system (Figure 1). When a physician considers motor neuron disease (MND), he or she must evaluate whether there is damage to the motor system; where the damage is and whether the damage involves the UMN, LMN or both pathways, and whether there is any indication of damage outside the motor system (which could indicate a diagnosis of something other than MND). A special test called the EMG-NCV (Electromyogram and Nerve Conduction Studies) is also necessary to help to detect damage to the lower motor neurons and exclude more treatable diseases such as motor neuropathy with multifocal conduction block (**See Table 1 for the classification of motor neuron diseases and Table 2 on differential diagnosis).**

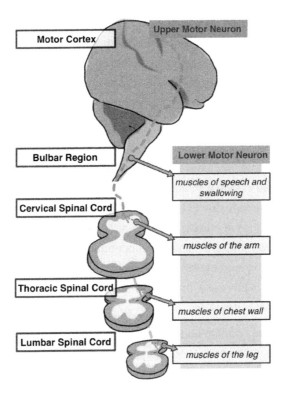

Figure 1: The motor system is comprised of an upper and lower motor neuron pathway that brings messages from the brain to the muscles.

Symptoms of damage to the UMN include stiffness, cramps, slowness of movement, laughing or crying too easily (termed pseudobulbar affect), nasal, slow speech, and sometimes the urgency of urination. The signs of upper motor neuron damage on exam include an increase in muscle tone or stiffness with resistance to movement called spasticity, increased reflexes (when the knee, ankle, inner elbow and arm are tapped with the reflex hammer), and abnormal reflexes (this includes an increase in chin move-ment with a tap called a jaw jerk, the presence of a Babinski sign where the big toe goes up instead of down when the sole of the foot is stimulated, and the presence of increased finger flexion on the appropriate stimulus).

Symptoms of LMN damage include weakness, thinning of the muscles or atrophy, twitching of the muscles or fasciculations, and cramps. The examination demonstrates weakness and atrophy with fasciculations and a decrease in tone with absent or diminished reflexes. The EMG will demonstrate damage due to LMN loss in the weakened muscles and may also show changes in muscles that are still strong. NCV studies should be normal; however, these studies are important because they help to detect motor neuropathy with or without conduction block in people with mainly LMN damage. In this case, these individuals may have a form of motor neuropathy that is treatable.

It is very important to understand that the presence of motor neuron damage does not mean that someone has ALS or any other motor neuron disease. A physician will rule out other causes of motor neuron damage before diagnosing ALS (Table 2).

Table 1: Classification of Motor Neuron Diseases

- UMN:
  - Primary Lateral Sclerosis (PLS)
  - Bulbar Palsy variant of PLS
  - Familial Spastic Paraparesis (Aut Dominant, X-Linked)
- LMN:
  - Spinal Muscular Atrophy (SMA)
  - Progressive Muscular Atrophy (PMA)

- Monomelic Amyotrophy (one extremity with slow progression)
- Brachial Amyotrophic Diplegia (progressive weakness of both arms with no bulbar or respiratory involvement)
- Kennedy's Disease (x-Linked Recessive)
- UMN and LMN:
  - Amyotrophic Lateral Sclerosis (ALS)
    - Sporadic
    - Familial ALS
  - Progressive Bulbar Palsy

Table 2: Differential Diagnosis of Motor Neuron Damage

A. Pure LMN

    a. Spinal Muscular Atrophy

    b. Progressive Muscular Atrophy

    c. Inflammatory Neuropathies

        i. Chronic inflammatory demyelinating polyneuropathy (CIDP)

    d. Motor Neuropathies

        i. Multifocal Motor Neuropathy with Conduction Block

        ii. Associated with tumors

        iii. Associated with metabolic problems

            1. Porphyria

            2. Gangliosidoses (including Tay Sachs Variants)

        iv. Associated with Toxins

            1. Lead

        v. Associated with Immune System Abnormalities

            1. Monoclonal Gammopathies and Myeloma

        vi. Associated with vasculitis

    e. Inflammatory Myopathies especially Inclusion Body Myopathy

    f. Polyradiculopathy due to degenerative spine disease

g. Electrical Injuries

h. Viral Infections

    i. Polio

    ii. Coxsackie

    iii. HIV

    iv. West Nile Virus

B. Pure UMN

a. Primary Lateral Sclerosis

b. Familial Spastic Paraparesis

c. Carrier of Adrenoleukodystrophy

d. Multiple Sclerosis

e. Mitochondrial Diseases

f. CNS vasculitis

g. Leukodystrophies

h. Brainstem lesions including syrinx, stroke, mass

i. Compressive cervical myelopathy

C. UMN and LMN

a. Amyotrophic Lateral Sclerosis

b. Spine disease

c. Nutritional deficiencies

    i. Vitamin B12

    ii. Copper

d. Vasculitis

e. Mitochondrial Disease

f. Toxins

    i. Mercury

g. Endocrine Dysfunction

    i. Thyroid and parathyroid

h. Neoplasms

    i. Lymphoma

    ii. Carcinomatous meningitis

Motor neuron diseases (MND) damage the motor system. They can affect either the upper motor neuron (UMN), the lower motor neuron (LMN), or both. These diseases are named for the part of the motor system they affect. In ALS, both the UMN and the LMN are damaged. Table 1 presents the classification of the more common diseases, listed by which portion of the motor system they involve. The classical MNDs include:

Amyotrophic Lateral Sclerosis (ALS) was originally described by Jean-Martin Charcot in the mid-1800s and is often called Charcot's disease in France. Classical ALS is a distinct syndrome characterized by a combination of UMN and LMN signs and symptoms without other neurologic problems and no other explanation but a motor system disorder. In approximately two-thirds of patients with ALS, the disease takes this classical form.

Progressive Muscular Atrophy (PMA) constitutes roughly 8-10% of patients with sporadic ALS. PMA is sometimes called Aran-Duchenne type of motor neuron disease (MND). The initial symptoms are manifestations of LMN involvement of the spinal cord and, in a later stage, of the lower brainstem. If UMN disease does not develop within two years, the disease is likely to remain PMA.

Primary Lateral Sclerosis (PLS) was first described by Erb in 1875. The clinical signs of PLS consist only of UMN signs. It is the rarest of all the forms of ALS.

ALS is a Motor Neuron Disease characterized by damage to both the Upper Motor Neurons and the Lower Motor Neurons. ALS affects people between 55 and 75 years of age although it can occur in individuals of all ages. The prevalence rate (how many people have the disease at one time) of ALS is about 4 per 100,000 people and its incidence rate (how many new cases occur in a time period) is about 1 per 100,000 new cases each year. There is also a male-to-female ratio of about 2:1.

The symptoms of ALS vary from one person to the next. Symptoms reflect weakness and thinning of muscles due to the involvement of the LMN as well as stiffness from the UMN involvement. Onset can begin in the muscles that are innervated by the bulbar neurons (speaking, swallowing) or in muscles innervated by nerve cells in the spinal cord causing weakness in one arm or one leg. In 20% of ALS cases, the ability to speak and swallow begin to decline first. In 80 % of cases, symptoms initialize in the limbs. A person newly diagnosed with ALS may trip, drop things, slur his/her speech, twitch, and laugh or cry uncontrollably. The person may also experience abnormal fatigue of the arms or legs and muscle cramps. Walking and activities requiring the hands may prove more difficult for a person with the disease. Over time, the disease spreads from one area to another and gradually, people living with ALS will lose movement in the muscles throughout their body, including the muscles that allow them to breathe. While the average lifespan for someone with ALS is about 36 months, it is important to recognize that 20% of people with ALS live for five years and 10% of patients live for ten years.

Recently, the medical community has begun to understand that in a small group of people with ALS, there may be frank dementia. This happens in only 5% of people with ALS. However, up to 40% of people with ALS do have mild cognitive involvement that may be evident on testing in the clinic.

Personal Reflection

By Latoya Weaver, PSC

Amyotrophic Lateral Sclerosis (ALS), also known as Lou Gehrig's disease, is a disease that until 2005 I had not known. It's amazing how quickly that changed when my mother was diagnosed.

Our saga started in 2005 at Drexel College of Medicine at the MDA/ALS Center of Hope where my beloved mother shared her symptoms of weakness in her arms and hands. At first it was surreal. I couldn't see how a twitch and some weakness in her arms could ever turn into full body paralysis and even death. My vibrant mother had ALS? Soon after her diagnosis, my family and I would notice each day how more and more of my mother's mobility faded. Years later, on March 2007, my mother made the difficult choice to be trached and ventilator dependent.

Once becoming ventilator-dependent, my mother's speech slowly faded away. Speaking is another function that we all take for granted. Have you ever wondered what would happen if one day you slowly started losing your ability to speak? My mother always talked, smiled and laughed, so her loss of speech was extremely hard for me. We went from being able to have a conversation, laughing, talking about anything our hearts desired to not being able to hear her say one word; her voice was gone. She could still make sounds and cry, but we would never hear her say "I love you" or anything else for that matter, ever again. We then relied on other forms of communication such as the EyeGaze communication system.

It's a good thing that the mind stays intact with ALS because my mother began to speak through her eyes. It took a while, but I came to master reading my mother's eyes. She just had to look at me and I knew what she wanted, or I'd hear a noise that she made, and I would know that she wanted a channel changed on the TV, or needed me to scratch her nose, or put socks on her cold feet.

ALS didn't stop progressing. It made my mother weaker and weaker, and slowly my mom progressed to the point where she was not able to move in bed at all. She went from sleeping in her own comfy bed to a hospital bed, and I went from being able to sleep in my own bed to sleeping on a folding bed beside her. If she needed suctioning or needed turning in bed, I was right there. My mother lost the ability to do something so simple that we all take for granted—sleeping. Turning over during sleep is something we all do on our own, but when you can no longer turn, then someone needs to help and I would get up and turn her over every two to three hours, just so my mom would not get any pressure sores.

Acceptance of my mother's ALS brought more love and appreciation to our family. No matter what hardship came our way, life was still full of love, happiness, joy, and meaning. God bless all who are and have been affected by this disease. Let's continue to speak loud and let the world know about ALS.

CHAPTER 2

Variations of ALS and Potential Causes

By Terry Heiman-Patterson, M.D.

There are both Sporadic (no family history) and Familial (family history) forms of ALS. Ten percent of people with ALS have a family history of the disease that has been identified as a genetic abnormality. 90% of people with ALS do not have any family history of the disease though it is now known that 10% of these sporadic cases do carry one of the genetic abnormalities described in Familial cases.

Sporadic ALS (SALS)

Sporadic or Classical ALS is a distinct syndrome characterized by a combination of UMN and LMN problems and occurs in about two-thirds of people with ALS.

Progressive Bulbar Palsy (PBP)

PBP was originally described by Duchenne in 1860. In approximately 25% of people with ALS, the initial symptoms begin in muscles innervated by the lower brainstem that control articulation, chewing, and swallowing. Sometimes the disease remains in this form for years, but usually it progresses to generalized muscle weakness, that is, to ALS. When the disease is strictly limited to the bulbar muscles, it is called PBP, not classical ALS.

Familial ALS (FALS)

In some instances, ALS runs in the family, i.e. it is familial and most likely has a genetic component. This happens in 10% or less of all people with ALS, although it is likely that genetic makeup may play a role in an individual's susceptibility to disease. A nice overview of genetics in laymen's terms can be found on the MDA website at http://www.mdausa.org/publications/gen_faq.html.

Familial ALS (FALS) cases comprise between 5-10% of all cases and is a dominantly inherited disease, meaning that one of the PALS' (Person with ALS) parents passed on the abnormal gene. Almost 20 % of people with FALS have damage (called a mutation) in the gene that codes for the protein Cu/Zn superoxide dismutase (SOD 1) located on Chromosome 21. To date, scientists have now identified more than 30 different genes that are either causal or increase the risk of developing ALS. In fact, the most common genetic cause of ALS is the abnormal extra chromosomal material in the C9ORF72 gene, called a hexanucleotide repeat. This abnormality has been found not only in 23% of families with ALS (Familial) but also in 5-7% of people with ALS and no family history.

Some of the genetic abnormalities can be present with either dementia, ALS, or both, underscoring the possible shared mechanisms in these diseases and the findings of cognitive involvement in people with ALS. It is expected that more genes will be found to be responsible for the disease through research and genetic studies in families and siblings of people with both Sporadic (SALS) and Familial ALS (FALS). These genetic changes will give us information about the pathways that are important for disease and lead to therapeutic strategies not only directed at FALS but also for SALS.

What are the Potential Causes of ALS?

The cause of ALS is not known. However, there are many pathologic mechanisms that may play a role in disease. It is likely that ALS is a complex multisystem disease with several mechanisms that cause the death of motor neurons. Any one of these mechanisms or a combination of several may be responsible for the disease, and many of these mechanisms also play a role in other neurodegenerative diseases. Furthermore, as pointed out above, there are likely to be genetic and hereditary factors that will modify the disease and susceptibility.

The most important potential mechanisms are listed below:

- Defective glutamate metabolism
- Free radical injury and oxidative stress
- Mitochondrial dysfunction
- Gene defects and RNA processing
- Programmed cell death (apoptosis)
- Cytoskeletal protein defects
- Autoimmune dysfunction
- Protein clumping and aggregation
- Toxic exposures

For descriptions of each mechanism, go to our Glossary of Terms in back of this book.

FYI: The National ALS Registry, a program to collect, manage and analyze data about persons with ALS, was launched in October, 2010 and is actively enrolling individuals with the disease. The Registry includes data from national databases as well as de-identified information provided by persons with ALS (PALS). All collected information is kept confidential. Persons living with ALS who choose to participate can add their information to the Registry by visiting www.cdd.gov/als

---

CHAPTER 3

Once Diagnosed:
Choosing the Right Doctor

By Dr. Terry Heiman-Patterson, M.D.

At the moment of diagnosis, people with ALS (PALS) and their loved ones begin a challenging journey that can be made less arduous with good medical care. The goal of good medical care must be to provide state-of-the-art multidisciplinary management of the disease, and also a haven for PALS and their families. When you look for a doctor, you are looking for an entire care team—one that will take this difficult journey with you, offering compassion and support as well as excellence in care.

The medical care team will include not only a physician but allied health professionals trained in the care of people living with ALS. This will include the Nurse Coordinator, who will screen for symptoms and support the physician in managing the symptoms medically. The Nurse Coordinator is usually the first person that PALS and their caregivers see regarding their issues and concerns. Other members of the multidisciplinary team include physical therapists, occupational therapists, speech-language pathologists, nutrition specialists, respiratory therapists, case managers and mental health support. While this sounds like a lot of medical staff, each professional plays a critical role in the care of a person with ALS. Multidisciplinary care has been advocated as a core measure in the quality care of PALS. In fact, it has been shown that not only is survival improved by the multidisciplinary approach to care, but so is quality of life.

However, while multidisciplinary clinical care is the gold standard, it is important to remember that PALS and their families come first! Each person is an individual and will have different preferences for their physician and care team. Some PALS may want a physician that is more paternal, making clear what decisions in care they would recommend, while other PALS may appreciate a collaborative approach in which information regarding care decisions is discussed, but decisions are left entirely in their hands. It is critical that PALS and their families seek out a physician that instills confidence in them while providing the style of care that is comfortable. PALS should be able to talk to their physicians with trust and openness. A chosen physician should demonstrate knowledge of ALS and a commitment to the disease, and should be a resource for research and information. He or she is the leader of the multidisciplinary team and will set the tone for the entire team. Remember that there will be important decisions regarding care and interventions, and a physician should be respectful of a patient's wishes.

While this sounds like a tall order, there are a large number of ALS specialty clinics across the country to choose from, as well as a number of caring neurologists. While the multidisciplinary clinic is ideal, an independent neurologist who is compassionate and caring may be able to identify local health care professionals who can fill the gap. The neurologist who made the diagnosis is a good starting point to begin your search for a long-term relationship and care team. The local neurologist may know of an ALS center, which can provide a second opinion and disease care. The local neurologist may also be willing to provide support or organize multidisciplinary help in conjunction or independent of an ALS center. This should certainly be considered if the PALS and family are more comfortable with the local neurologist. It would also be important to visit the closest ALS center to determine if this care is what you are comfortable with.

In order to identify an ALS clinic in your area, the first step would be to look at the clinics supported by the Muscular Dystrophy Association (mda.org) or The ALS Association (alsa.org). Typically, address and contact information is provided on these websites. Once you have identified a clinic or physician near you, the next step is to make an appointment at the clinic to determine if the visit provides you and your loved one with medical treatment and support that you find helpful. The visit begins with the first phone call and carries through the entire appointment.

When you think about what your family wants from a clinic visit and the care team that provides treatment, some of the important questions to consider include:

- *Was the support staff responsive to your telephone call?*
- *When you and your loved one arrived at clinic, were you made comfortable?*
- *Was the physician open and caring?*
- *Was the physician patient and thorough?*
- *Did the physician answer all your questions and provide information about the disease, treatment and research?*
- *Were the allied health professionals knowledgeable?*
- *Did the allied healthcare professionals address and answer your questions?*
- *Did you feel that the visit was helpful?*
- *Did the visit make you feel more hopeful?*
- *Did you feel this team would be accessible for follow-up questions?*
- *Was the philosophy of care in line with your own?*

If the answers to these questions are yes, your loved one may have found a home for his or her care. Remember that every person living with ALS is different, and every clinic will have its own ambience. It is important that the clinic can provide what the PALS and family feel is needed.

At the MDA/ ALS Center of Hope in Philadelphia, we consider the PALS and family the most important people in the room and encourage our PALS to seek care where they are most comfortable without regard for what they think might hurt our feelings. Our philosophy remains steadfast:

we wish to provide compassionate and knowledgeable care in a warm and safe environment. ALS is a family disease, and we at the clinic are the extended family. To that end, we wish for every person living with this disease a clinic that meets their own personal needs and stands ready to partner with them on the ALS journey.

For a list of ALS clinics in the United States, go to the Resources section of this book.

FYI: In addition to Lou Gehrig, former governor of Massachusetts, Paul Cellucci and former senator, Jacob Javits lived with ALS. Television contributors, Jon Stone and David Niven also battled ALS. Currently, former pro athletes: Steve Gleason, O.J. Brigance, and Kevin Turner are courageously battling ALS. They have all started nonprofits, so please see their work and missions in our Resources.

CHAPTER 4

How to Tell Family and Friends

By Mary Paolone, MSRN

Now that you have gained some information on how to connect with health-care professionals, let's discuss issues and suggestions related to sharing the news of ALS with family, friends, co-workers, etc. How you navigate this chapter will greatly rely on how you are coping with the knowledge of your loved one's diagnosis. Since going forward hinges on this detail, let us briefly address the various feelings that may be arising, as well as the different ways in which people manage these emotions.

Depending when your family learned of ALS, you may have already or may presently be experiencing a wide range of feelings, emotions, questions, and considerations. We often explain to our new families that it may feel like a rollercoaster of emotions, as your reactions and thoughts race in all directions. Be prepared that for a while you may feel more intolerant of situations, your sleeping and eating may be affected, you may be more tearful at times, your motivation and interests may decrease, and/or you may want to be alone more often. These and other experiences can certainly be normal responses to learning of ALS. It can be helpful during this time of adjustment to be patient and gentle with yourself and others, as you integrate this new information into your life. However, if these situations do not balance out after a period of time (everyone's timing is different), and the negative emotions begin to outweigh the positive, we would encourage you to speak with your physician or nurse about options for additional help; such as counseling, support groups, books, stress management, medications, etc.

If you are more of a social person and were raised with an ease of communicating, then you may be more likely to seek the support of others. On the other hand, if you grew up in an environment where you did not feel comfortable sharing your feelings and thoughts, or are more of an introvert, then you may have more difficulty. Most important is the idea that neither of these approaches is right or wrong, better or worse, and there are certainly many other ways of managing adversity. It is, however, how we meet challenges that can certainly make our journeys easier or more difficult. That is why it is helpful to understand how you normally react and cope, figure out if this coping method is helpful for you, and decide what may be best for you going forward. Be aware of your own feelings and emotions as much as you can, and use tools such as journaling, talking, movement, spiritual support, counseling, meditation, etc. if/when needed. Once ALS has entered your life, stress is a constant factor, so learning how to handle it will take you far. If you have difficulty handling the stress, be sure to seek help from a coach, doctor, friend, counselor, or spiritual advisor.

Now that we have briefly addressed how you and your loved ones may be coping with the diagnosis of ALS, think about how you might tell others about the diagnosis. As we mentioned before, this conversation depends largely on how you are managing all of this, so please take your time and move at your own pace in sharing the news. Some concepts we will consider are: when to share the news, who to share it with and how to go about doing so.

As mentioned previously, when you tell others about your situation depends on your own personal approach and your own acceptance of the diagnosis. If you rush to explain what is happening before you have at least an understanding of the disease itself, misinformation could be relayed, leading to more distress for everyone. On the other hand, if you wait too long, some people may become confused or frustrated if they sense that something is wrong. Generally speaking, there is no wrong or right time to discuss the news of diagnosis, and sharing this information with others can only increase your network of support when moving forward.

Now, let us look at who to tell. This too is a personal decision. Are there people who live with you or see you on a daily basis, such as family? Co-workers? Friends? They will probably notice physical changes. If this is the case, it may be much more difficult to keep the diagnosis to yourself. It is certainly not necessary that you divulge all the details of your situation if you do not wish, but sharing some general information about your diagnosis with your loved ones and the people with whom you have daily contact is probably most beneficial.

So now we will discuss the tricky part—what to say and how to say it. Much of this will again be determined by your own level of comfort as well as who is receiving the information. If you are speaking with co-workers, you may want to consider scheduling a meeting after work hours. Let your boss know that someone you love is battling ALS and describe the disease and the toll it takes. If your role as a caregiver limits your ability to work, it can be helpful to discuss your options with your Human Resources Department.

There can be several nuances for divulging news of a terminally ill loved one at work, depending on your specific situation and job duties. We encourage you to seek counsel and support from your ALS team if you anticipate difficulties in communicating your situation within your work environment.

It's best to encourage and model ongoing, open and honest communication with your confidants. Be prepared though that not everyone knows how to or is capable of dealing with the emotional and physical changes that ALS will bring along. Take value and appreciate those that support you. Also try to understand and accept those who are not comfortable being a part of the ALS journey.

When having the discussion with other family members and/or friends, rely on your intuition, as you know those people and situations best. It is an uncertain time for all involved, so the more support, clarity, and compassion you can offer during these conversations, the better.

Good To KNOW: The more you know, the more tools and resources you will have available to you as the disease progresses. Go to the American Disabilities Act site at www.ada.gov and learn about Patients' Rights.

Personal Reflection

By Jodi O'Donnell-Ames

It is not something most of us think we will have to do, and I wish you didn't have this situation or responsibility. At some point, you will have to explain to your child or grandchild that someone he or she loves has ALS. I had the conversation with my daughter, Alina when she was four years old and it was one of the hardest things I have ever done. Alina had many questions. She listened and processed the information the only way her four-year-old brain could at that point and went off to play Barbies. As my late husband Kevin's illness progressed, so did her questions and to this day I regret that I was not fully honest with her.

The day before Kevin passed; I said everything except that Daddy was going to die. I said that Daddy was very sick; Daddy wouldn't be here, etc... I could not say the words myself, so how could I have said them to her, my precious child?

However, years later, Alina told me that she was not prepared for that day, and I wish I had had the courage to say those words. Alina was eight years old when Kevin passed, and all I wanted to do was protect her. Knowing that she was a very mature and verbal eight-year-old, I should have better prepared her for such an enormous loss.

I did the best that I could and you will too. Somehow, you DO find the strength.

Good To KNOW: Several popular books about ALS which can be shared with family and friends are:

Tuesdays with Morrie by Mitch Albom

I Remember Running: The Year I Got Everything I Ever Wanted and ALS by Darcy Wakefield and Jonathan Eig

Until I Say Good-Bye: My Year of Living with Joy by Susan Spencer Wendel and Bret Witter.

Additional books can be found in our Resources.

It's a great idea to share a brochure, book or website about ALS with those who want more information and invite questions and discussions to keep open and honest communications.

CHAPTER 5

Starting a Gentle Conversation with Young Children

By Mary Paolone and Jodi O'Donnell-Ames

There is no easy way to tell a young child that someone they love has been diagnosed with a scary, life-threatening disease. Since we cannot take this burden away from you, in this chapter we hope to offer some ideas/suggestions that could potentially soften the task a bit. Most importantly, you know your child/children and family dynamics best, so trust your intuition and inner guidance as you move forward. There are many things to consider before you begin this type of conversation, so please take your time to make sure that it is an appropriate time for everyone involved.

Consider the following ideas and questions to ensure the best possible outcome for all:

- Have you been crying or does anyone feel/appear upset?
- Do you feel prepared/able to manage and support your children during the discussion?
- Did everyone get enough sleep?
- Did everyone eat?
- Is there enough time for all of you to talk, be heard and comfort one another?

• Who is going to be with you to support you during this conversation?

Before you begin, consider your child's age and level of understanding and maturity. You may want to start with your older children first. We often suggest some pre-planning of what you may say or the words you may use in talking with your children. Many parents discuss this very topic with the mental health specialist at their clinic. If your schedule permits, allow sufficient time to talk about ALS and avoid rushing the process or discussion, which could lead to negative fallout later. Remember, there is no "perfect" time for a conversation of this nature, although you can make it as good as it can be with some preparation, planning, patience and a lot of LOVE.

Here are a few ways to begin.

Using a resource can be helpful for younger children. Find an age-appropriate book and read it together. We have suggested books according to age and they can be found in our list of Resources. Starting the discussion with a book or prop can help to create a focus for everyone. Depending on the child's age, snuggle and read out loud or read together as a family.

You may want to begin by asking your child his/her thoughts about the parent's or relative's current symptoms, which can lead into a fuller discussion of the facts. Other options may be something like these statements: "As you have noticed, Daddy has been having difficulty walking, and after so many doctors' appointments, we have finally learned why." Or, "I have not been feeling well lately and have finally received a diagnosis and reason why I have been falling." It can be helpful to name the illness and share a few facts about it with your child (considering his or her age). If you can, share a positive outlook or fact about the illness to introduce hope (e.g.—"I have a great team of healthcare professionals to help us."). Know that your child will often follow your lead in how this challenge is presented and managed.

Invite an open and honest conversation. Let your child know that he or she can ask questions, even though you may not know the answers. Tell them that even if they do not wish to discuss it now, they can come to you at any time. Most importantly, reassure the child's security and basic normalcy despite the changes that may occur. Discuss what may change (Mom helping Dad more or vice versa/helpers in the house), and what will stay the same (the child going to same school/schedule/house, etc.). Do this to the extent that you're able to be honest and again, be age-appropriate with the amount of information given. Children tend to have less anxiety when they can expect what is to come.

As you know, children are all very different and therefore, may react very differently to this news. Some children become quiet and withdrawn, while others may act out and behave differently. Still others might feel guilty in some way, thinking somehow that ALS is their fault. In the months that follow this discussion, try to be aware of changes in your children, and why those changes may be happening. Notify teachers, school counselors and child-care providers about what is happening in your family, so they can be aware and act as resources if needed.

Older children may ask about their roles as helpers. Although it may be difficult to verbalize that you may need help, know that this can be a valuable lesson about life. When times are tough, many families come together and work together as best they can. On the same note, do not force a child to help if possible. Suggestions and ideas can be planted, but allow your child to come to the decision to help on his own. Aim for balance. Children can be part of the helping team, but they also need to have fun and be allowed to be kids.

Overall, and as we stated in the beginning, you know your children and your family best. The suggestions offered here come from years of personal experiences and have worked with many families dealing with illness and change. Use which suggestions feel right as well as the resources listed, and most importantly, trust your intuition!

Good To KNOW: MANY schools now provide support groups for children. Ask your child's school if they have a support group that would be appropriate and helpful to your child as he or she watches and experiences a parent or loved one battle ALS.

Personal Narrative

By Nora Ames

Although I run the risk of sounding cliché, I think of my mom, Tina Singer Ames, often. She passed away just eight months after being diagnosed with ALS when I was nine years old, and I have now lived more of my life without her than I did with her. As such, I have had many important milestones to reflect on- I thought of her as I shopped for my prom dress, when I graduated high school, then college, when I passed my boards to become a nurse, and when I rented my first apartment on my own. She will be on my mind when I get married someday and tell my own children about their grandmother, and she remains with me now. I have thought often about what kind of person my mom was, who she was as a person, what she wished for me, and how my life would be different if I'd never heard of ALS.

Over the years since she passed away, I have tried to form my own image of her, as it turns out, with some difficulty. After all, your impression of your parents when you are nine years old is far from crystal clear; all I knew at that age was "Mom," I had yet to know "Tina" at all. As I have gotten older and heard stories of her pre-"Mom" life, the more I know that I love Tina just as much as I loved Mom. As I became a caregiver to her when she was struck with ALS (however limited that role was as a nine year old child), our roles were somewhat reversed. She was still Mom, but now *I* helped *mom* get up the stairs, *I* wiped off *Mom's* face, *I* helped *Mom* put her shoes on. All of a sudden, I went from being a child whose biggest concern was who I was going to trade snacks with at school to a child who was forced to grow up too fast. It was a role I dove into headfirst and took very seriously (at least in my nine-year-old mind). I took on the role of caregiver wholeheartedly, even after my mom passed away, feeling that I needed to be a surrogate mom to my younger brother.

As I look back, I simply wish I had had more time. I never got the chance to know my mom as anything other than Mom, and it is one of my biggest wishes in life to have been able to know her as Tina. So for those suffering with ALS, I urge you to let your kids know who you are. Embrace the changing roles, let your kids help (trust me, it makes them feel special!); but most of all, let them know you as a person. Even if they are too young right now, leave letters for them to open on important milestones, leave them notes, leave them pictures, leave them stories. Tell them about how you met their dad/mom; tell them about yourself as a child; tell them about what clique you belonged to in high school; tell them about the crazy things you did in college! Above all, just let your children know you beyond your role as their parent. Your kids, no matter how young, will think of you for the rest of their lives, in all of their important moments, so give them lots to remember.

Nora Ames

Nora is a tireless volunteer at Hope Loves Company® and MDA. She's a nurse by profession and enjoys baking, reading, and traveling. She and her brother Adam are the inspiration for the book, **What Did You Learn Today?**

FYI: Nora's experience is not unusual. Many times, in the midst of crises, recording memories is not a priority and understandably so. If you have the means, hire a professional or ask a talented friend to help preserve memories in scrapbooks, take biographical videos and record letters or journals as keepsakes.

CHAPTER 6

What Kinds of Treatments Are There for ALS?

By Terry Heiman-Patterson, M.D.

While there is no cure for ALS as of this writing, there are available treatments including medicines and interventions, directed at the symptoms as well as the disease.

There is one medicine, Rilutek, which slows the disease progression by decreasing glutamate levels. Also, there are many ongoing clinical trials that use agents that target possible causes of the disease. Furthermore, advances in the aggressive treatment of breathing problems in ALS with noninvasive ventilation and respiratory management, as well as aggressive nutritional intervention, have provided significant improvements in survival and quality of life. Finally, there are symptom-specific treatments and interventions that are best implemented in a multidisciplinary approach that has led to improved quality of life and maximization of function in people living with ALS.

In the multidisciplinary setting, physicians work in tandem with a team of healthcare professionals skilled in the care of people with ALS. The team typically includes nurses, nutritionists, occupational therapists, physical therapists, speech and language pathologists, mental health specialists, and case management professional. These professionals will help to identify problems as well as provide solutions while working together to maintain the individual's function and mobility along with his or her overall quality of life. The role of each clinic team member is outlined in Table 3.

The only drug approved to specifically treat ALS as of this writing is Rilutek. Studies show that Rilutek helps to protect nerve cells from damage by reducing the amount of glutamate in the nervous system. It is important to understand that Rilutek will not restore any loss of function prior to the start of treatment. It only slows the progression of these symptoms. The recommended dosage for Rilutek is 50mg (one tablet) every 12 hours. The medication should be taken at the same time every day, both morning and night and should be taken at least one hour after meals. The most common side effects of Rilutek are weakness, nausea, dizziness, headache, and elevation of liver enzymes. If there is nausea, a doctor may recommend that the medicine be taken with meals. It is not recommended that individuals smoke or drink excessive amounts of alcohol while taking this medication, as smoking may decrease the amount of Rilutek in the bloodstream and alcohol may contribute to elevated liver enzymes and may cause an increase risk of liver problems.

The key to selecting possible therapeutic agents lies in the understanding of the disease. To date, the cause of ALS is not known but several theories have been proposed, and there is experimental evidence to support each theory. There may be an interplay of one or more of these mechanisms that lead to nerve cell death in ALS. Furthermore, there may be genetic factors that are important to the predisposition to develop disease with the right provocation. The mechanisms of neuronal death in ALS that have been theorized include: defective glutamate metabolism, free radical injury, protein aggregation, mitochondrial dysfunction, gene defects, programmed cell death (apoptosis), cytoskeletal protein defects (including neurofilament abnormalities), and immune system dysfunction. These proposed causes of ALS have provided targets for drug and stem cell therapies. Several resources for finding updated information regarding enrolling trials are available including:

MDA.org, http://www.als.net/ALS-Research/ALS-Clinical-Trials/, ALSA. org, http://www.alsconsortium.org/and clinicaltrials.gov.

While there is no cure for ALS at present, there is treatment. Clinical management of ALS is focused primarily on symptom relief. Treatment of symptoms increases the quality of life for people living with ALS by reducing complications and increasing comfort. Furthermore, aggressive respiratory and nutritional intervention can improve both the morbidity and mortality that result from ALS.

The most common symptoms in ALS include muscle cramps and stiffness, increased salivation and drooling, increased secretions with thickened phlegm, constipation, depression and anxiety, increased laughing and crying called pseudobulbar affect, fatigue, and insomnia. Less frequently, people with ALS may have urinary urgency and throat spasms. There are many strategies including physical interventions and medicines available to treat the symptoms that are associated with ALS. Table 4 lists some of the commonly used physical interventions and medicines.

Table 3: Multidisciplinary Team Members

Team Member	Role
Neurologist	The neurologist will help to diagnose your disease and direct care throughout the course of your illness. The neurologist will see you at your clinic visits and identify changes in function and direct symptom management.
Nurse Coordinator	The nurse coordinator acts as your liaison or "go-to person" anytime you have questions or needs. While at the clinic, the nurse coordinator helps to ensure that all of your issues are addressed with each team member. After your appointment, your Nurse Coordinator will assist you with questions, medication renewals or any problems or concerns that arise between your visits.
Mental Health Specialist	The role of the mental health specialist is to provide counseling to you and your family. She is also available to other healthcare providers as a consultant on the psycho-social dynamics of ALS and can recommend strategies for the identified concerns.

Physical Therapist	The physical therapist will address mobility issues including walking, transferring from one place to another, and getting in and out of bed. Recommendations to optimize the performance of these activities will then be made based on the findings. Assistive technology is also discussed to help optimize independence.
Occupational Therapist	The occupational therapist will concentrate on areas of self-care (such as dressing, feeding, bathing, grooming, etc.), work and leisure activities. Use of adaptive devices or techniques will be recommended as appropriate. The occupational therapist works along with the physical therapist to evaluate home accessibility; wheelchair specifications and provide caregiver education.
Speech and Language Pathologist	The speech language pathologist will monitor the status of your speech and swallowing ability. Suggestions will be provided to ensure maximum effectiveness in communication. Alternative or augmentative devices will be introduced and reviewed as you may need them. Safe swallowing techniques and possible diet modifications will also be discussed.
Nutritionist	The nutritionist will assess your nutritional status by discussing your current diet, challenges with eating or digestion, and weight changes. It is critical that you maintain proper nutrition in order to feel your best. The nutritionist may recommend diet modifications that will enhance longevity and quality of life, such as using thickened liquids, eating softer or chopped food, and alternative modes of nutrition such as a feeding tube.
Respiratory Therapist	The respiratory therapist will perform an assessment of your respiratory muscle function including PFTs (pulmonary function test) and examination of your breath sounds. The therapist will also address some issues with noninvasive ventilation and clearance of secretions, working closely with your physician to optimize your ventilator status.
Case Manager	The case manager will advocate on your behalf and help you with your individual, medical, or insurance needs. The case manager is able to coordinate appropriate services ordered by the physician, such as home physical therapy, occupational therapy, nursing, respiratory therapy, and hospice care.

Research Coordinator	The research coordinator is available to disseminate information about current ALS studies and provide further information to interested individuals. They will screen prospective participants, conduct the study sessions with those individuals who meet the criteria, organize data and medical records, and communicate with other research staff throughout the country as indicated.

Table 4: Treatments for Common Symptoms in ALS

Symptom	Physical Interventions	Medicines
Cramps	Positioning, stretching, massage, pool therapy	Magnesium 400-600mg/day, Vitamin E 400iu 2-3/day, Clonazepam, Baclofen, Zanflex, Dilantin, Tegretol, Gabapentin, Pregabulin
Anxiety	Counseling, biofeedback	Lorazepam, Ativan, Paxil, Buspar
Constipation	Fluids, fiber, fruit	Dulcolax, Milk of Magnesia, Colace; Miralax, Lactulose
Phlegm and thick secretions	Hydration, suction machine, coughalator, vest, cut back on dairy	Guaifenesin, nebulizer treatment
Depression	Counseling	Antidepressants including SSRIs (Sertraline, Paroxetene, Citalopram, Escitalopram, Fluoxetine), SNRIs (Venlafaxine),and others (Bupropion, Mirtazapine)
Increased Secretions and Drooling	Suction Machine	Atropine, Glycopyrrolate, Scopolamine transdermal patch, Hyosciamine, Amitriptyline, Botulinum toxin, radiotherapy ablation
Dry Mouth	drinking extra fluids, review medications	

Twitching or Fasciculations		Baclofen, Neurontin
Fatigue	Rest	Amantadine, Methylphenidate, Amphetamine and Dextroamphetamine combinations, Pyridostigmine If breathing problems contributing with increased CO_2 then NIPPV (noninvasive ventilator or bipap)
Emotional Lability (laughing or crying too easily)		Neudexta, Sertraline, Amitriptyline
Laryngospasm		Baclofen, Diazepam, Omeprazole
Sleep disturbance	Sleep hygiene	Amytriptyline, Trazodone, Chloral Hydrate, Diphenylhydramine, Lorazepam, Temazepam, Ambien If respiratory problems contributing NIPPV
Stiffness (Spasticity)	Range of motion, stretching, massage, pool therapy	Tizanidine, Baclofen; Dantrium, Diazepam, Botox injections
Urgency	Toileting schedule	Oxybutinin

FYI: There are ALS clinical trials taking place around the world. For more information and a list of trials, go to ALS Therapy Development Institute's site at http://www.alstdi.org/als-research/als-clinical-trials/, to NEALS (Northeast Amyotrophic Lateral Sclerosis Consortium); http://www.alscon-sortium.org/clinical_trial_news.php and https://www.clinicaltrials.gov/

CHAPTER 7

What Is Adaptive Equipment and How Can it Help PALS?

By Sara Feldman, PT, DPT, ATP

Changes in muscle strength lead to changes in the way people do their everyday activities. Often, adaptive equipment will assist a person with ALS in performing his or her activities throughout the day. The equipment may be new to you or your loved one, but it is familiar to the multi-disciplinary clinic team of rehabilitation therapists, which will include physical therapists (PT), occupational therapists (OT), and speech-language pathologists (SLP). Their roles are to follow the PALS throughout the progression of the disease to help maximize his or her safety and function. Physical therapists use assistive devices that will enhance mobility, assist with the completion of activities, or maximize safety and independence. Similarly, occupational therapists use adaptive equipment that will aid in the completion of daily living, work, and leisure activities. Speech-language pathologists work with equipment for communication. An assistive technology professional may deal with all of these issues. Below are the many types of adaptive equipment that may help to enable individuals with ALS to function as independently as possible:

Assistive Devices for Mobility

Assistive devices to aid in walking may be the first recommendation given to those with ALS. To determine the need for an assistive device, a PT will measure the strength in the PALS' legs, trunk, neck, and arm, as the strength in these areas affects mobility. They will assess an individual's range of motion, looking for tightness or lack of flexibility at the joints. Also, they will test balance and coordination and ask about any history of falls as well as the person's activity level. It's important to be honest with your PT and OT at your visit so that they can best meet your needs as well as your safety.

A single point cane is often the first device used for someone with balance issues. At first, it may be needed outdoors and on uneven surfaces only. It will provide a touch point to help maintain balance; it is similar to the balance provided by resting a hand on a wall or dresser. Some people find it more comfortable to use two canes to maintain their normal gait pattern, but others may choose to use forearm crutches if they need this level of support. If more support is necessary, a walker is advised. Due to the extra work required to pick up a standard walker, a PT will most likely recommend a rolling walker. The basic model looks like a standard walker, but with wheels attached to the front. Usually, the rear rubber caps need to be covered, or replaced with a material that can slide easily on a variety of surfaces. Rollators are similar to rolling walkers and provide excellent support but require less work to use. The main difference is that they have a seat that allows a person to sit if he or she needs to take a break and rest. Both models fold down for easier transport. Occasionally, a walker with extra support for the arms is recommended. This is a platform walker and can be somewhat large and unwieldy, but may offer enough support to help maintain an upright position and allow an individual to walk independently longer.

Understandably, the decision to use a wheelchair is difficult; however, this could mean deciding between going places or staying in one place. There are two types of wheelchairs, manual or power. A manual wheelchair is propelled by either the individual or a caregiver. Power wheelchairs are battery powered and are controlled with joysticks or switches. The lightest styles of manual wheelchairs have four small wheels and fewer removable parts. These types are known as transport, companion, or travel wheelchairs. Often the armrests, and sometimes the footrests, are part of the frame. They have good transportability because they are lightweight and fold easily. That said, they are difficult to use on uneven surfaces, and if sitting in the chair, the only way to move it is by using one's feet. Standard or lightweight manual wheelchairs have a larger rear wheel, permitting movement of the chair with those wheels. The armrests and leg rests often swing away or are removable. These wheelchairs fold for transport, but they are heavier than the transport chairs. A therapist may recommend a seat cushion since the seat itself offers no pressure relief. Custom features can be added to improve the fit and support of these chairs. There are also models that offer tilt or recline options to change the position of the back if the person has weak trunk or neck muscles.

For more independence and increased mobility, power options are preferable. Power scooters may be appropriate for a specific time period if there is trunk, head and arm strength, but limited leg strength. Insurance companies often either do not cover power scooters at all or will not cover a power scooter with a progressive diagnosis. If this device is more suitable for the PALS, he or she should look into other ways to buy the scooter. Power wheelchairs are the primary means of mobility for many people with ALS when walking becomes too difficult. These customized, multi-function wheelchairs provide not only a means of getting around the environment but also allow the adjustment of one's position while in the chair. These custom power wheelchairs require an evaluation by an assistive technology professional and can take weeks or months to acquire, so a conversation with a therapist and neurologist about power wheelchairs is recommended as soon as walking difficulties begin.

Orthotics

Based on the evaluation of a therapist and a neurologist, it may be rec-ommended for the individual with ALS to utilize leg braces to assist with walking. This loss of motion, specifically in the ability to lift one's toes up while walking, can be due to weakness or increased tone. Bracing helps to keep the foot in proper positioning while walking and swinging through with a leg and putting a foot down on the ground. Over-the-counter braces, such as an ankle brace or posterior leaf splint, may offer enough support initially. High top shoes can also offer some ankle stability. If more support is necessary, custom molded ankle foot orthotics (MAFOs) that are custom fabricated to meet the individual's needs are recommended. Articulating, or jointed, MAFOs are the most commonly prescribed brace as they prevent the motion of the foot dropping down that should stop, but still allow for passive dorsiflexion when needed. Carbon composite braces offer a lighter weight option and are becoming more widely used. If more stability is necessary, double upright metal bars with attached shoes or solid ankle orthotics may be an appropriate recommendation. Braces are most often up to the height of the calf, but it may be necessary to use a brace above the knee. They may be used alone or with one of the assistive devices such as a cane or a walker, and can be prescribed for either one or both legs.

Stair Climbing

Climbing stairs can become difficult if a person is experiencing weakness, because in order to use stairs, one's full body weight needs to be lifted up and down. A railing or banister is suggested on one side at least, or both, if possible. If the rise is too high, it may be possible to make modifications or convert the steps to a ramp. The standard coding for ramp accessibility is one foot of run for every inch of rise. Personal residences do not need to meet that standard, but for safety, the measurements should not be less than ten inches of run for one inch of rise.

Another option for negotiating the stairs is to get a stair glide, which is a chair that travels up the stairs on a track. A stair glide may be purchased or rented; however, the cost varies according to the length and direction the track must take. The most expensive, but sometimes only, option is to install an elevator between floors. This is the best option if travel between floors in a power wheelchair is desired.

Bed Mobility

The first concern of the day for someone with ALS may be how to get in and out of bed. If there is difficulty with moving in bed, adding a grab rail to pull on or a footboard to push on may be enough. A bed rail can be added by attaching it to the metal frame, or using a sliding one, attached to a board between the mattress and box spring. There are also "ladders" made of rope or canvas that attach to the frame and lay on the bed as something to pull on to help with turning. Flannel pajamas on flannel sheets can make turning extremely difficult; so, consider smoother satin sheets for easier sliding. Using a wedge under a pillow to remain partially raised can make sitting up easier. If these solutions are unsatisfactory, consider a hospital bed. Fully electric beds provide a wide range of motions such as raising and lowering the head, the feet, and the overall bed height. Put the electric bed side-by-side with a twin bed to imitate a double bed. Insurance companies tend to cover the semi-electric beds that don't raise up and down electrically. Commercial adjustable beds are also available. Some issues with commercial beds include their lack of ability to be raised and lowered, their weight, and the inability for a transfer aid to be positioned underneath on some models. However, they may still be an option considering an individual's circumstances.

It can be quite difficult to find the right mattress for a bed. A person with ALS should consider what it is about a mattress that he or she does not like in order to examine which options best suit his or her needs. If it is too soft, perhaps adding a board under the mattress can help to make it firm. If it is too hard, then consider adding an overlay mattress. There is no one size fits all for mattresses, and insurances will only pay for gel overlays or air mattresses if someone has already experienced skin breakdown. Changing positions may be helpful either by using the features of the bed or having someone assist. One way to make it easier for a caregiver is to use a draw sheet, which is a sheet put between the individual and the bed sheet. Pull on the sheet to slide the patient up or down, side-to-side, or assist turning to one side.

Transfer Aid

Transfers refer to moving from one place to another or from one surface to another. For example, going from a sitting position to a standing position is a transfer. If this is becoming difficult, it is recommended to choose a seating arrangement where the hips are higher than the knees. Raising seat heights with a pillow or block of foam may be beneficial in this way as well as choosing firmer seats and seats with armrests that enable more leverage than would otherwise be possible. There are also devices that can help lift a person up from his or her seat. One device sits on the seat and uses hydraulics to raise or lower you slowly. This can be quite helpful if an extra push is needed to get up. They are not designed to be sat upon for long periods or helpful once standing. There are also recliners that include a motor to not only lay an individual back, but also help to stand him or her up. Insurance will sometimes help pay for the motor piece if the individual is still ambulatory, but not for the chair itself.

If someone is helping an individual with ALS to stand, he or she should be mindful of his own body mechanics and speak to a therapist about appropriate techniques. Using a transfer belt around the waist may help give a caregiver a place to hold on to rather than pulling on the person's arms. If the individual is able to stand with assistance, but his feet are often caught up during the turning part, a pivot disc may be of use. Similar to a Lazy Susan, it is placed on the floor and allows a caregiver to turn the individual while he or she is standing on the disc. If standing is too difficult, but the individual has trunk and arm strength, a transfer board could be a better option. The board is placed partially on the surface being transferred from, and partially on the surface the individual is being moved to. This builds a bridge between the two places and allows movement safely across.

If none of these are options, there are mechanical lifts that will assist a caregiver. The most common is a sling style lift. The individual can sit on a sling that is attached to a device that has a boom that can be raised or lowered. Some of these are electric, but insurance plans frequently pay only for the kind that a caregiver will have to pump. Once in the sling, the device moves from place to place with the individual in it. There are other styles that assist with stand pivoting, but they generally require some trunk control and can be uncomfortable if the individual cannot tolerate pressure on his or her chest or stomach. The barrier-free style lift also requires the use of a sling; however, the sling attaches to an overhead track, alleviating the need for the device to be moved across the floor. Many caregivers find this style much easier to use though the track distance is limited.

Typically, bathroom equipment and items to assist with activities of daily living (ADLs) are addressed by the occupational therapist. To determine the need for an assistive device, the OT will measure arm strength, and will also take into account trunk, neck, and leg strength, as all of these can affect an individual's ADLs. They will assess the range of motion specifically to identify any tightness or lack of flexibility at the joints, as well as test balance, coordination, and gross and fine motor skills. They will ask about work and leisure activities and an individual's activity level.

Bathroom Equipment

The bathroom is a key area of focus for occupational therapists and a primary area of concern for many people. It is a small space where the surfaces become slippery when wet. Moreover, people with ALS may not be using their usual braces or assistive devices while in the bathroom due to space constraints. This combination leads to the need for increased safety awareness. One place to start may be with non-skid strips or a bath mat on the floor, or the individual, and the caregiver can wear non-slip water shoes. Adding grab bars in the tub, shower area, and by the toilet adds to safety. The configuration of the bathroom will determine the best places to install the grab bars.

A shower seat or tub transfer bench can make showering safer and save energy. The addition of a hand-held shower attachment makes showering easier, too. Additional helpful items include a long-handled sponge/bath brush for washing the back and feet, a bath mitt for holding the soap and washcloth, and pump dispensers for shampoo and soap. The safest, most accessible, option is to have a completely barrier free shower, with no lip at all and use a roll-in shower chair. These chairs are made of PVC pipe with a mesh seat and back, and can be wheeled from the bed to the shower and over the toilet.

If the toilet is difficult to get on and off, options include adding arms via a frame around the toilet, raising the seat height with seat attachments, and using a commode or shower chair. A bidet is a toilet or toilet attachment that aids hygiene by washing and drying after using the toilet. They can be stand-alone fixtures or attached to an existing toilet bowl. There are also devices that are used to assist with holding toilet paper.

Activities of Daily Living Tools

There are various kinds of tools or devices available to assist with the activities of daily living associated with grooming, hygiene, dressing, cooking, eating, work, and leisure activities. A general rule that may assist individuals with ALS in being independent is to use large handled items or adding padding, such as foam or pipe insulation, to enlarge handles on frequently used items. For example, padding can be added to the handle of a toothbrush or razor, or electric versions of these can be use as they tend to have thicker handles. If gripping becomes difficult, a universal cuff may be best. If the individual's arms get fatigued or are weak while managing activities, he or she can try sitting and propping them up on a table or arm supports.

Assistive devices for ADLs can be found online or in stores, and a clinic therapist is the best resource in this regard. Other solutions include an electric toothbrush, hair dryer holders, long-handled hairbrush, electric razor, modified nail clippers, long shoe horn, sock-aid, elastic shoelaces, zipper pulls, buttonhooks, Velcro, larger handles, utensils, universal cuff, and rocker knife.

Communication Devices

The SLP will evaluate speech and swallowing function and make recommendations based on his or her findings and the individual's preferences. Communication devices range from low-tech letter boards to high-tech eye gaze tracking, computerized speech generating devices. There is a place for both types of devices, and a low-tech letter board should always be available for times when a computer-based system is impractical. The first step many people find useful is to write notes, and this can be done on a basic notebook or electronically. Tablet computers provide the option of speaking what is written. A letter board is paper, often laminated, with the alphabet on one side and frequently used expressions on the other. They can be customized to the person and can be made small enough to be worn on the sleeve or large enough to be on a wall. The letter choices are made through direct selection, a person can point either at the letter, or through a scanning method where someone points at the rows, then columns until he or she reaches a choice. Another type of letter board, the E-tran, has the alphabet written around the outside in the six quadrants. A two-step method can be used to look at the group of letters, and then through a space cut out in the center before looking again to indicate which position the letter is in. The electronic version, the MegaBee, uses a similar two-step method with position and color indicating the letter and the caregiver types the letters out as they're spelled. Alternately, the letters can be written on a clear piece of Plexiglas so the individuals can look at the letter from opposite directions until their eyes meet.

Tablet computers and iPads can also be used as AAC (Augmentative and Alternative Communication) devices and are becoming the first option people try. The text- to-speech apps range from free of charge to costing as much as $200, and offer a variety of ability levels. Basic apps provide basic text to speech, while the most advanced apps resemble the software on speech generating devices. The free ones are usually not recommended because they have limited voice options and ads. If typing on the virtual keyboard becomes difficult, then it is possible to add switch access to the tablets, but usually the Speech Language Pathologist will discuss other communication options. These options include computer based AAC devices. These high-tech SGDs work along the continuum of abilities, thus allowing access to them with hands, a mouse, a switch, and all the way up to EyeGaze. They provide additional features including computer access and environmental control.

Computer Access

Computer use has become important for both work and leisure. Difficulty accessing the computer can stop individuals with ALS from using one, even though computers can help them stay actively connected to the outside world. Issues with computer access usually progress concerning an individual's difficulty using the keyboard, mouse or both. If the individual is experiencing weakness in the shoulders or elbows, supporting the forearms or lowering the keyboard or mouse may be helpful. If there is weakness in the wrists or hands, using wrist supports or typing aids may be an appropriate assistive measure.

Computers also have accessibility features built into their operating systems that allow PALS to change certain settings to make the keyboard or mouse easier to use. These can be found under the Accessibility section in the Windows operating system and Universal Access on a Mac. Commonly used keyboard features are the on-screen keyboard and Sticky Keys. With the on-screen keyboard, the mouse can be used to move the cursor across a keyboard on the screen to type. With Sticky Keys, the function keys are held down until the next key is typed. Early changes to the mouse features include changing mouse styles, changing the size and speed of the cursor, or using a head or foot mouse. If making selections via clicking becomes difficult, external switches can be added or clicking programs can be downloaded, such as Dwell Clicker, which allows the user to make the selection just by hovering over it. Another alternative for some people is to use the voice recognition features of the computer or add a program such as Dragon Naturally Speaking. Often a mix of techniques will be used as needs change. The highest tech option is to use an EyeGaze tracking device to move the cursor with a dwell click option. These are typically found on speech generating devices, but can also be purchased as separate products.

For individuals with ALS, the use of adaptive devices and techniques may mean the difference between being able to complete an activity or not. There are many options available and the therapists at a multidisciplinary team clinic will be able to discuss these options in detail to help determine the best choices for each individual.

Good To KNOW:

Dressing can be made easier by choosing clothes with elastic and Velcro instead of buttons, zippers and laces. Consider using ponchos instead of coats and slip-on shoes versus those with laces. Modifying clothing you already have is also an option. Replace buttons with Velcro; cut shirts up the back so you slip them on from the front rather than overhead; replace regular laces with elastic laces; etc.

CHAPTER 8

Should Children Be Involved in ALS Care?

By Mary Paolone and Jodi O'Donnell-Ames

If a child of any age wants to be helpful, YES!

Allowing children to participate in the care of a loved one grants quality time, fosters a nurturing nature and positive self-esteem. However, no child should be forced into being helpful. Allow children to determine if they are comfortable with helping, and to what degree. Young children are natural helpers. They love to help and feel proud when tasks are accomplished. Even the smallest of children can get daddy's slippers or mommy's sweater.

ALS can rob patients of strong voices or voices at all. If that's the case, allow the child to choose books and read to the parent or relative. Reading out loud together is a great way to learn and grow and, of course, snuggle!

When it comes to older children, follow their cues. Children who are forced to be caregivers might do so with frustration or resentment. If and when children want to help with caregiving, allow them to decide how they will help. If they are not sure how they can help and ask for advice, the following ways are some suggestions (Please note that tasks will vary based on age and maturity levels):

Household chores

Some provide more enjoyment than others. For example, making dinner can be a fun way for children to chip in. Accept what has been prepared and show appreciation. Dinners may not be as good as mom's or as nutritious as preferred, but preparing a meal is one more thing crossed off the list of things to do, and the helper will gain valuable life skills. Children can also help with dishes, laundry and pet care.

Hands-on care

Some children or young adults are natural caregivers and may want to provide hands-on care. If everyone is comfortable with that, it's a priceless gift of nurturing and reciprocation from child to parent and can be beautiful. Hands-on care needs depend on the patient's stage of illness, and how many caregivers are involved. There are numerous ways to provide hands-on care without getting too personal. These may include assistance with eating, grooming (nails, hair), and dressing (socks and shoes), etc. How is it possible to know if or when a child is comfortable with hands-on care? Watch. When comfortable, he or she will most likely jump in to help. That's a good starting place for everyone involved.

Secretarial

Some young adults are very organized and would rather delegate and facilitate jobs. If they feel so inclined, they can make phone calls and coordinate the care of their loved ones. This is a great way to be involved on a peripheral level for children who aren't comfortable with hands-on care. Children also love to use their computer skills. They can also help to type schedules and send emails.

FYI: Theoretical Physicist and Cosmologist Stephen Hawking, who has ALS, has lived 50 years since his diagnosis. The story of his journey with ALS was captured in the recent Academy Award-winning movie, *The Theory of Everything*.

Personal Narrative

When My Normal Teenage Life Was Flipped Upside Down

By Mackenzie Anderson

No matter how much I try to forget the dreary, August night in which my parents came home from yet another hospital trip, I cannot. That night, out of the 5 months of searching for a reason why my mother's left index finger drooped just a little more than all of the others, turned out to inform me that my worst fear had become my new reality. My mother, only 50 years old at the time, had been diagnosed with a fatal neuromuscular disease, ALS. *"How did this happen?"*, I remember asking myself. Most kids normally wouldn't have even been familiar with the disease and what it encompassed.

However, after months of endless hospitals tests, my dad and I decided to look up potential diagnoses on our own time. While researching online, I got bored and logged into Facebook. To my surprise, there was what seemed like hundreds of videos posted of my friends partaking in the ALS Ice Bucket Challenge.

Curious as to what the disease entailed, I "Googled" it and the results made my jaw drop. The symptoms for the disease were almost a complete match to what my mom had been experiencing, and although my dad originally shut down my hypothesis, claiming that mom had to have an illness with a cure, I knew somewhere deep down that I was right. I knew that no matter how much I wanted to trust my dad that everything would be okay, that this wouldn't be the only time we would talk about ALS. *Why now?* I remember wondering.

Fast forward only 11 months later and my mom no longer has any use of her hands, is in a wheelchair almost full-time and will be having a feeding tube put in next month. The reality of this overbearing disease is that I had to grow up faster than any 17-year-old should. Also, thousands of children who have a parent or grandparent with ALS, some even younger than myself, are placed in this same position. Feeding, toileting, and bathing become an ingrained everyday task that we are accustomed to doing, without question. Although, the physical tasks are not even the worst part of the disease. The most difficult part of the experience has been the mental strain. I have had endless days of wondering: *How did this happen? Why now? Why my mother? Why me?* But the conclusion to which I have finally arrived at is that as much as ALS has changed my life for the worse, it has also allowed me to find my true self, my true friends, and my true passion.

After my mother's diagnosis, I was tired of sitting around and acting sorry for myself each day. So, I decided to be proactive. Since then, I have raised over $27,000 for the ALS Association and received an internship at my local ALS chapter. These new opportunities have helped me to discover what kind of person I want to be in life and what really matters. For me, this includes making my family my number one priority, having a couple close friends who really care about me and steering clear of all unnecessary drama (including drugs, alcohol and even, some people). Nonetheless, one of the greatest things that this disease has done, and yes I meant to say the greatest, is that it has helped me to develop relationships with those who have a direct connection to someone with ALS. These people have helped me to stop asking "why?" and, instead, have taught me to ask "how?". How can I help find a cure? How can I help others cope with the diagnosis? How can I make a difference in this world?

At some point after deeply struggling with my mother's fate, I allowed myself to reach out for help—something I used to detest asking for. After trying to speak with my friends, guidance counselor and even a therapist, I still felt as though no one could truly understand how I was feeling or what I had to deal with on a day-to-day basis. So, I decided to search for a support group for children and found Hope Loves Company® and their Camp HLC®, a camp for kids affected by ALS. This small group of people has become some of the best friends I could have ever asked for. Simply knowing others who are able to relate to the situations which I am going through, is extremely comforting. I strongly encourage any teen or child who has a parent or grandparent with ALS to find either a support group or attend "Camp HLC®" (or BOTH), as it helps you to know that you truly aren't alone.

Caregiving for someone with ALS may be one of the most difficult things in the world, and attempting to do so as a child may seem downright impossible. However, with the right people by your side, the right mentality, and the right environment, the impossible can become achievable. Just remember that asking for help can only make you stronger!

Mackenzie Anderson

Mackenzie is a high school senior who lives in Foxborough, MA. Her mother was diagnosed with ALS in August of 2014 and since then, Mackenzie has been a dedicated ALS volunteer and advocate. In addition to her work for the ALS Association, she is the President of her school's DECA chapter, President of Community Warriors (a community service club), and Publicity Coordinator of Spanish National Honor Society. Also, Mackenzie will be awarded her Girl Scout Gold Award this fall, which is equivalent to being an Eagle Scout. In college, Mackenzie aspires to study business and use her degree to better the world, in one way or another.

CHAPTER 9

Parenting and ALS

By Jodi O'Donnell-Ames

An ALS family is a unique family. Although roles may change, and challenges are many, love and support are the constant thread in holding an ALS family together. Never underestimate a child's role in that unity. As a certified teacher, I have worked with children for most of my life. I have also raised three children who have lost a parent to ALS and understand how complicated life becomes for everyone in the family when a parent is ill. With that in mind, I have included a few suggestions below that were helpful to me as I learned to balance parenting with caregiving. Be patient with and aware of the organization and teamwork required for this juggling act.

Getting Help

People living with ALS need support. Caregivers need support, and so will other family members, especially children. Be sure to let schoolteachers and counselors know what your family is facing. Patients and caregivers will have less time to be parents. Be sure to ask trusted family and friends who have children of a similar age to include your child on fun excursions. Allow your child to be a child and enjoy playdates and outings.

Additional Helpers

A trusted relative or friend who does not have children can also be helpful. He or she can provide special bonding time such as a day at the beach or amusement park, and the one-on-one time may provide an opportunity for your child to share feelings about the situation. Encourage the adult to listen to the child, but not to necessarily bring up the family situation on each and every outing. Sometimes your child may just need time to do ordinary things without thinking about what is going on at home. For those family members with children, please invite the children of PALS on fun excursions. When travel became challenging, I sent a letter out to our family and friends and asked if they could include Alina in their plans, especially during the summer months. We wanted our child to have fun, but I was torn between taking care of my husband and taking Alina to the park. Knowing that our child has a fun day out while we were at the doctor's office eased our minds.

Special Reading Time

Try to find uninterrupted, quiet time to read an ALS children's book with your child (see Resources) or have him or her read it to you. Be patient and allow enough time for questions, and answer those questions to the best of your ability. Listen closely and you will learn what he or she already knows. Remember that young children often want to hear the same information, or the same story read to them, more than once. Be patient and allow them to choose a favorite or new book that relates to the PALS' illness as often as they would like. As they grow and learn, they may have new questions, or need more complex answers to the same questions.

When You Can't Be There

When one parent is ill, the other parent must divide his or her time. When you can't be there in person, find creative ways to remember your child. Leave notes in hiding spots or in lunch boxes, or buy and wrap a small surprise to place under the pillow. Make a video of family memories that your child can view while you are at the doctors or hospital. These small gestures will guarantee smiles for sure!

Involve Your Child

If a child expresses an interest in caregiving, allow it. Helping is a form of affection and may provide feelings of pride and accomplishment. The reverse is also true. A child may be uninterested in caregiving. Don't make your child responsible for taking care of a parent in ways he or she is not yet ready for. Allow the parent to be a parent and the child to be a child as much as possible.

Pay Attention

Kids cope and grieve differently. Some children may become withdrawn while others may get angry. Think before you react to your child's behavior. Was there another change in the PAL's condition? Did Mom just get a feeding tube? Did another PALS acquaintance lose his battle and your child overhear the news? Remember that although your child may not talk about what's happening, that doesn't mean it's not helpful to do so. There may come a time when counseling support will be helpful. Let your child know that it's ok to seek and receive professional help.

Love Your Child

Showering your child with love, whether you are the parent with ALS or the caregiving parent, is the most important thing of all. Forming great memories of love and affection are healing for the entire family. Document those memories on camera and video. If you have the energy and strength, write love letters to your child for special occasions down the road. These will certainly be cherished.

Good To KNOW: Author Jodi O'Donnell-Ames and her late husband Kevin wrote cards for each of their daughter Alina's milestone events. Even though this was very difficult to do emotionally and physically in the midst of ALS (Jodi read Kevin's lips to write his sentiments), the cards have been priceless gifts for Alina over the years.

Personal Narrative

How My Dad (Kevin O'Donnell) Parented From a Wheelchair

By Alina O'Donnell

After being diagnosed with ALS, many typical parent-child activities will become difficult, and then impossible. My dad could never coach me in sports (which is perhaps why I'm so athletically impaired), swing me around, or give me "airplane rides" like my friends' dads could. He could, however, personally chauffeur me around the neighborhood in his wheelchair- one that went 7 miles per hour, and that was pretty cool. Here are some of the other ways in which my dad and I embraced his wheelchair in new traditions.

Play Board Games

My Dad and I spent hours playing our own, slightly adapted version of chess. To this day, I don't know the real rules of the game. When he lost the ability to use his hands, he would tell my mom where to move the pawns. Of course, he also indulged my competitive edge with Candy Land, Monopoly and Chutes and Ladders.

Invent Wheelchair Games

This can include your own! I was lucky to grow up in a house with a big, sprawling backyard. My dad and I loved to play hide and seek, though I must confess, sometimes I cheated and followed his wheelchair tracks.

Bake Together

If I'm being honest- the extent of our baking was a concoction we dubbed "Waffle Supreme." The foundation, a fluffy Belgian waffle, was always the same. The toppings varied according to what junk food we had readily available- ice cream, gummi bears, potato chips, you name it. Note: Waffle Supreme makes for a nutritious and satisfying breakfast, lunch or dinner.

Play Computer or Video Games

This is one activity that no Generation Z child will protest. My dad introduced me to and nurtured my addiction to a "Lion King"-themed computer game. Always the computer master, he would show me different shortcuts and cheat codes. I also loved to sit on his lap and watch him play Deerhunter, much to my mom's objection.

Watch a TV Series Together

The three of us, sometimes joined by a handful of relatives and close friends, watched Survivor every Thursday night. To heighten the excitement, we placed bets on who would be voted off that episode and even threw a few singles into the pool. I loved this weekly tradition, which also served as an excuse to eat popcorn, watch PG-rated reality TV and stay up an hour past my usual bedtime.

Offer Online Homework Help

My father was diagnosed with ALS in 1994, the advent of the Internet's popularity. At just six years old, my math skills were already embarrassingly stunted. Once a week, he would force me to watch tutorials and take online practice tests. This was back when homework was done solely by the (now obsolete) pencil and paper.

Take Videos

My parents slept in the wheelchair-accessible downstairs, which meant I had the entire second story of our house to myself. You can probably imagine what this looked like—a colorful mess, strewn with blanket forts, toys and books. When my dad could no longer walk upstairs, my mom took videos of me reading and playing in my hand-painted room so that he could feel like he was there with me.

Even though my dad lived with ALS and our situation was different, my time with my father was appreciated and enjoyed as much as the next daddy's girl!

Alina O'Donnell

Illustrator of *The Stars that Shine*, one of the few ALS children's books available. *The Stars that Shine* is based on Alina's experience as a little girl when her daddy Kevin battled ALS. Alina works for the City of Philadelphia and enjoys writing, running and traveling.

CHAPTER 10

ALS and Prolonged Care

By Terry Heiman-Patterson, M.D.

Remember that each person is different and the choice of medicine to be used is best determined by the treating physician. Careful attention to swallowing and feeding is also important, and aggressive management should be initiated to avoid aspiration (food entering the windpipe) and weight loss. If swallowing problems (dysphagia) are present, the speech-language pathologist (SLP) should educate the person living with ALS about the appropriate food consistency and proper swallowing technique using a chin tuck. Additionally, the patient should sleep with his or her head elevated and should never lay flat following meals. A physician, along with a speech and language pathologist, may recommend a video swallow evaluation to assess the risk of aspiration. As swallowing difficulties worsen, or if vital capacity (a pulmonary function measurement) drops below 50%, a percutaneous gastrostomy (PEG) tube should be recommended to maintain nutrition. This is a small tube inserted into the stomach during endoscopy and requires only sedation without general anesthesia. While the PEG tube will improve nutrition and reduce the risk of aspiration, it does not fully prevent aspiration. Early intervention with PEG tube can prolong life.

Breathing trouble is another symptom that must be managed by those with ALS. Normally, the lungs function to allow a person to breathe in air (oxygen) and exchange it for carbon dioxide, a waste product of metabolism in the body. This exchange takes place in the air sacs called alveoli. During inspiration, which is an active process, air is drawn into the mouth, down the large airway called the trachea, and then into the bronchi, and finally into the smaller airways (bronchioles) to the air sacs (alveoli). The exchange of oxygen and carbon dioxide takes place in the air sacs or alveoli, and carbon dioxide is then expired out of the lungs through the passive process of expiration. The diaphragm and chest muscles (called intercostals) are responsible for inspiration and the abdominal muscles and other chest muscles (the internal intercostals) help with expiration.

In individuals with ALS, several problems cause difficulties in breathing. First, as the respiratory muscles weaken, oxygen cannot be adequately exchanged with carbon dioxide which then builds up in the blood stream. This leads to sleepiness and fatigue. Furthermore, since the respiratory muscles are weak, there is a decrease in the strength of the individual's cough. A weakened cough and a decrease in gag reflex lead to problems clearing the airway and mouth of secretions. As swallowing difficulties progress, oral secretions increase as a result. These secretions can get into the airways and alveoli, blocking the adequate exchange of oxygen. The decrease in effective coughing further compromises the ability to clear those secretions. Finally, if the muscles in the back of the throat are weakened, the airway is unprotected when the individual swallows. This leads to aspiration, where the contents of the oral cavity can enter the person's airways. Aspiration can lead to infection (aspiration pneumonia) as well as the further compromise of carbon dioxide exchange. Additionally, with increased swallowing difficulties, oral food intake is reduced, and malnutrition occurs. Malnutrition leads to further compromise by increasing overall muscle weakness including the respiratory muscles.

The symptoms of respiratory failure, which can be a serious issue for an individual with ALS, include shortness of breath during exertion or at rest, fatigue, inability to sleep flat, troubled sleep, daytime sleepiness, yawning, and morning headaches. The examination may show rapid breathing, the use of extra muscles to help breathe, problems with speaking including low volume and frequent breaths, along with an ineffective cough. If aspiration is also a problem, there may be coughing with eating, watery eyes, sneezing, alterations in breathing, changes in lung sounds, gagging, frequent throat clearing, swallowing more than once for each bite or sip, and even a gurgly sound to the voice. As respiratory failure worsens, there can be a buildup of carbon dioxide, which results in sleepiness and confusion,

In order to combat these symptoms, in addition to asking about symptoms that indicate respiratory muscle weakness, a doctor can measure the muscle strength and function in the clinic using a machine called a spirometer. The amount of air that the lungs can hold is called its vital capacity (VC). Similarly, the strength of inspiration (breathing in) and expiration (breathing out) can be measured with a small pressure gauge. Most centers measure the vital capacity at a baseline and with each visit. As the vital capacity decreases or symptoms occur, measurement of the oxygen and carbon dioxide levels in arterial blood can be performed. Furthermore, as the level of the vital capacity drops to half that of a normal set of lungs (50%), consideration should be given to the initiation of non-invasive positive pressure ventilation (NIPPV). NIPPV is a machine that pushes air into the lungs through a mask or interface. The person using the machine then breathes the air out against a lower pressure. This helps to keep the air sacs open.

The treatment for breathing problems in individuals is as follows:

General assessment

Physicians will generally perform a baseline examination and pulmonary function testing as well as assess any other medical conditions that might contribute to respiratory problems, including asthma, COPD, and congestive heart failure. Risk factors, such as cigarette smoking, secondhand smoke, dusts and fumes, and exposure to people with acute viral respiratory illness should be identified and avoided. Pneumovax immunization and yearly influenza immunizations are advised. Respiratory symptoms along with pulmonary function testing should be performed at every visit to allow early intervention and treatment of respiratory problems. As part of the routine care of people with ALS, physicians should aggressively treat acute respiratory infections, manage secretions, and institute noninvasive ventilation at the appropriate time.

Since acute respiratory infections can precipitate respiratory failure in a person who already has muscle weakness due to ALS, leading to invasive ventilation with intubation, (i.e. putting a tube down the mouth into the airway to help with breathing), infections must be treated aggressively. The additional secretions combined with an ineffective cough and reduced strength of the breathing muscles lead to increased secretions obstructing the airways. This further reduces the exchange of carbon dioxide and oxygen and resultant elevated carbon dioxide. For this reason, individuals with ALS may need to be in the hospital even with a mild upper respiratory infection to allow for intravenous hydration, antibiotics, and aggressive secretion management.

As mentioned earlier, increased secretions, whether from an acute respiratory infection or the inability to swallow properly, combined with re-duced protection of the airways from a weakness of the protective muscles oropharynx or poor cough, leads to a plugging of the airways, collapse of the air sacs, and infections secondary to aspiration. These all result in increased carbon dioxide as well as reduced oxygenation of the blood. Treatments are directed both at decreasing and thinning the secretions as well as increasing clearance. Medicines that decrease secretions include Anticholinergic medications (Glycopyrrolate, Amitriptyline, Transderm Scopolamine,Levsin or Hyoscyamine), and a botulinum toxin injection into the salivary gland. If these modalities fail, irradiation of the parotid gland can be helpful. If the secretions are thickened, especially with the use of anticholinergic agents, hydration, Guaifenesin, Propranolol, Acetylcysteine, and nebulization treatments can also be considered.

A doctor should recommend a program to promote the clearance of secretions when PALS can't do so independently. One of the interventions that can help is the use of an assisted cough machine (coughalator). If secretions are thick, a nebulizer may help along with chest percussion either manually by cupping the hands and tapping the back in different positions or through a mechanical vest that can help to mobilize the secre-tions. If the cough is weak, an assisted cough or coughalator can help to bring secretions up and, if necessary, a suction machine can be used to clear the mouth when the secretions are brought up. Using an incentive spirometer at home may help prevent airway collapse. In addition, the use of a medicine called Theophylline may improve diaphragmatic function and cough.

Use of noninvasive ventilation in ALS

As the deterioration of muscle strength and respiratory function caused by ALS progresses, the need for ventilatory assistance should be considered. In recent years, nocturnal noninvasive positive-pressure ventilation (NIPPV) has become the treatment of choice for patients with chronic respiratory insufficiency due to ALS. The noninvasive ventilator is triggered by the patient's own breathing and reduces the work of breathing, improves the exchange of carbon dioxide and oxygen, and improves sleep quality. Furthermore, it has been shown to prolong survival as well as improve the quality of life in people with ALS who are able to use it regularly. Other beneficial effects of NIPPV in patients with ALS include improvements in their overall quality of life and their cognitive functions. This includes measures of fatigue. Presently the accepted recommendation for starting NIPPV is an FVC (forced vital capacity test) of 50% expected or symptoms of respiratory failure (shortness of breath, daytime sleepiness, etc.).

Invasive Ventilation

As ALS progresses, the person living with the disease may become increasingly dependent on ventilation and, ultimately, will require invasive ventilation with a tracheostomy (tube placement into the main breathing pathway, the trachea, through the neck.) This will provide more efficient ventilation and better control of the upper airway and secretions. The decision to proceed with tracheostomy and invasive ventilation is often difficult and is highly individual. During the decision-making process, there must be an ongoing educational program that includes the person living with ALS and their family and caregivers, along with healthcare professionals, as the decision can certainly change. As the person living with ALS considers whether to choose a ventilator program they should understand their insurance coverage, family support, their level of independence, and financial resources. The choice of a home ventilation program requires supportive families and 24-hour supervision by family members and nurses.

Withdrawal of Care

If a person who is on a ventilator program decides that he or she would like to terminate ventilator support, a careful and thoughtful approach is necessary. There needs to be a complete discussion of the decision to terminate care and the ramifications of such action. Counseling to assure that the person understands the decision and treatment of depression is important. Once the decision is finalized, palliative care and sedation should be initiated as the ventilator is titrated off. Comfort care should be attended to by the physician throughout the process.

Personal Reflection

Kevin's Choice to Use a Ventilator

By Jodi O'Donnell-Ames

I will never forget the day that Kevin chose to be vented. At the time, his breathing capacity was at 35% and he was relying more and more on a Bi-Pap machine. Our daughter, Alina was six years old and he was struggling with how to proceed in his ALS journey. Kevin gave deep consideration to every decision he ever made. He was a man who made lists of pros and cons and he prided himself on his precision and accuracy of detail. While his body was failing him, Kevin was a young father and husband who lived life to the fullest and had many goals in mind. There were things he wanted to do before he left this earth and finally, after several days of sleepless nights and deep contemplation, Kevin told me that he was going to be vented. We cried and hugged and I immediately grabbed a notebook. Together, we listed the things he wanted to do with time on his side and the ability to have a machine breathe for him. Those next few days were euphoric-filled with renewed hope and plans.

Our list looked like this:

- **Go to the movies**
- **Go to an Eagles game**
- **See Alina receive her first Holy Communion**

- **Take Alina to a museum**

- **Renew our Vows and have a BIG party**

Being ventilated did mean more time and memories for Kevin and our family and everyone who loved Kevin was glad to have him with us longer because of his decision. Being ventilated does give you more freedom on life, but less freedom in other ways. For us, it also meant more help in our home, more equipment, backup equipment and NEVER leaving Kevin unattended to make sure his vent was working properly.

It also meant being more creative (Kevin lost his ability to speak after being ventilated) and we learned to communicate by reading his lips and then later with the help of his communication device. Also, we learned a new way to shower Kevin (with a machine in tow) and to travel with the necessary medical supplies. But we soon adjusted and enjoyed the plans that Kevin made when he decided to be vented. I know I speak for everyone in our village that we were so happy that Kevin chose to be ventilated and continued his fight with ALS.

CHAPTER 11

It Takes a Village

By Jodi O'Donnell-Ames

After years of being a caregiver to my late husband Kevin, I coined the slogan, "*Because if you live with ALS, so does your family.*" By that I mean that everyone involved and helping is affected by life with ALS. As your loved one becomes increasingly dependent, those closest to him or her may fall into caregiver roles. Everyone can help in some capacity; having a strong village means **more quality** time with your loved ones. The following chapter will help you to prepare, accept, assemble and maintain a team of helpers.

Accepting Help

As word of an ALS diagnosis spreads, people will ask, "What can I do to help?" At first, you may have difficulty answering this question. Accepting help means opening your door to others and inviting them in to witness and share a scary and emotional passage with you.

In our six- year journey caring for Kevin, the volunteers and helpers who stayed the course shared three common traits: gratitude, positivity and resilience. They relished their time with Kevin, especially when he thanked them through his speech device or said, "I love you" with his eyes. Trust that volunteers are grateful for the chance to be with you and your family and to be of help. I was once told that if I denied volunteers the opportunity to help, I was denying them of Kevin's time- time that was precious to those who loved him.

One resource that we personally found very useful is the book: *Share the Care: How to Organize a Group to Care for Someone Who Is Seriously Ill* by Cappy Capossela and Sheila Warnock. What Cappy and Sheila have done is to use their combined experiences and what has worked for them and implemented those successes into a book. This resource includes the steps involved in providing long-term care for a loved one and the paperwork to get things started. You can find their book and website in our Resources.

My sister-in-law Keiren Dunfee ordered the book, "*Share The Care*" and then implemented the program in our home for us. It was one of the best gifts Keiren could have given us! With the help of our STC team, we had volunteers bring meals, run errands to the grocery store and pharmacy, supply assistance with Kevin's range of motion and evening routine, home maintenance, lawn care and much more. It was a wonderfully organized and well-oiled program that gave us hope and rejuvenation on difficult days.

Assigning Help

The most helpful tasks are those that allow you to spend more uninterrupted time with your PALS. When you are a caregiver, the most trivial day-to-day chores are often neglected. Create a list of chores that need to be attended to on a weekly basis and make it readily available to those who offer help by sharing copies. This will enable you to assign willing caregivers jobs that meet their skills and levels of comfort. Maintaining caregivers over long periods of time will be easier if they enjoy their roles and feel appreciated as well.

Running Errands

ALS families, especially those without a wheelchair-accessible van, can't just get up and go. Brainstorm a list of all the errands you typically run in a week- the grocery store, bank, pharmacy, post office, library, etc.

When you think of something you need, jot it down on a notepad so that you can allocate responsibilities as efficiently as possible. Most neighbors will be heading on errands anyway, so, adding a few items to their list is acceptable.

Dinner Delivery Rotation

When you are too overwhelmed to prepare dinner, you should seek volunteers as needed. Provide a list of family favorites and special needs. Is your PALS able to eat? Which foods can he or she eat? Does your son have a peanut allergy? You may be uncomfortable with providing food recommendations or dietary restrictions, but remember that these details are necessary to ensure that the volunteer's time and food is not wasted. Years later, we still laugh about our lasagna dinners. Many kind, well-meaning neighbors brought lasagna to our door during Kevin's sickness. As grateful as we were, there is only so much lasagna one small family can eat!

Childcare

For young families with PALS, please ask your community of volunteers to help with your children. People living with ALS need support. Caregivers need support, and so do children. Be sure to let schoolteachers and counselors know what your family is facing. Patients and caregivers will have less time to be parents. Be sure to ask trusted family and friends who have children of similar ages to include your child on fun excursions. Allow your child to be a child whenever possible.

Additional Helpers

A trusted relative or friend without children can also be helpful. He or she can provide special bonding time such as a day at the beach or amusement park, and the one-on-one time may provide an opportunity for your child to share feelings and concerns. Encourage the adult to listen to the child, but not to necessarily bring up ALS on each and every outing. Sometimes your child may just need time to do ordinary things without thinking or worrying about what is going on at home.

Correspondence

Organized volunteers who enjoy paperwork can be very helpful keeping track of bills, cards, appointments and medication schedules.

Home and Yard Maintenance

No matter what time of year, there are external and internal chores to maintain a home. Handy persons can help with cleaning and organizing inside and lawn care, repairs outside. Knowing that entropy is not wreaking havoc on the home will lend a peace of mind to both PALS and CALS.

Massage and Physical Therapy

By all means, if you are fortunate enough to have a friend or family member who is a massage or physical therapist, don't hesitate to ask for help for both you and your loved one with ALS. In my opinion as a licensed massage therapist, massage is an extremely helpful modality. One simple explanation is that human touch is powerful. Emotionally, touch helps to decrease fear, loneliness and pain. Physically massage helps to increase circulation, flexibility and endorphins while decreasing heart rate, blood pressure, and stress.

Good To KNOW: The book, *Share the Care: How to Organize a Group to Care for Someone Who Is Seriously Ill* by Cappy Capossela and Sheila Warnock, also has a wonderful website. http://sharethecare.org/. Go right to the direct source for your caregiving needs at http://sharethecare.org/caregivers-concerned-friends/. Share it with other CALS and caregivers.

CHAPTER 12

Embracing Your Role as Caregiver

By Jodi O'Donnell-Ames

"Caregiving often calls us to lean into love we didn't know possible."
Tia Walker

While being a caregiver is profoundly rewarding, it can also be exhausting, frustrating, and depressing. Watching someone you love battle, ALS is a tragedy. Knowing that he or she can live and cope with ALS because of YOU is a gift.

I have found the following words to be helpful reminders in all aspects of caregiving: patience, acceptance, trust, commitment, flexibility, compassion, and respect. Both care provider and receiver should do their best to keep these words in mind.

Once, at 3:00 am in an ambulance during one of Kevin's many trips to the hospital, I met a dedicated young EMT whose reverence I will never forget. He said, "I treat every patient like my grandparent." His powerful words have remained with me for more than a decade. I think of him and his mantra whenever I am called to help someone who is ill.

Caring for the Caregiver

Caregiver burnout is common. I don't know how many times I was told, "If you don't take care of yourself, how can you take care of Kevin?" However, I still ended up in the hospital because of exhaustion twice. Do not let this happen to you!

Aside from a salary and a degree, there is little difference between a professional nurse and a volunteer caregiver. Just like overworked nurses, caregivers must learn how to refuel their furnaces. Most caregivers go from working a standard, 40-hour workweek to caregiving 24/7. To avoid crashing, you must find time to eat and sleep well, to relax, play and laugh when possible. I must admit, twelve years after Kevin passed, his private duty nurse and our Hope Loves Company® board member Lynne Brosche recently shared this quote with me. "In all of my years as a nurse, Jodi was very much an exception as far as a caregiver. I never knew anyone who slept in the same bed as their PALS and who gave care side by side with the professional nurse. Most family caregivers take a respite when the nurse arrives."

Aside from Lynne's quote, my dear friend Allison reminded me recently to share this with other caregivers as to not set impossible expectations and to tell you honestly what happened to me after YEARS of never leaving Kevin's side. I remember the first time that Kevin gave permission to his nurse to complete his morning routine which consisted of personal hygiene, meds, stretching, feeding, vent care and dressing. It was only months before Kevin passed and his nurse asked Kevin if it would be ok if SHE handled his morning routine and thus gave me a break. I was standing bedside and Kevin lifted his eyebrows in approval.

"Are you sure?" I asked Kevin. Again, his eyebrows raised. This meant two things to me: Alina was at school and safe and Kevin was in good hands as well. I, however, had three hours and had NO idea how to spend those three hours. I had given up everything. With the exception of being a compassionate caregiver, I no longer did the things that made me who I was. The only thing I knew was loving and caring for Kevin and I had no idea how to respond to this free time.

I was told to go and have fun so I got into my car and drove. I drove in anger and in tears. I had three hours to spend on a life that no longer existed. After driving, crying, walking then running, I came home and napped. Perhaps, that was what I needed to do with my time. While I felt compelled, almost obsessed with Kevin's care, it's best to continue a space for you, a moment to connect outside of ALS, somewhere in each busy day.

Nutrition

Make sure you get your protein and stay hydrated. It's a good idea to eat small meals throughout the day to keep your energy up.

Sleep

Whenever you have the chance! No one understands the relevance of sleep until it is no longer a privilege. Lack of sleep wreaks havoc on the body. It causes weakness, cloudy thinking, poor decision-making, headaches, limited patience, anxiety, and depression. If good a night's sleep is not an option, nap when a nurse or additional caregiver arrives.

Me Time

Although you might think it's selfish and impossible, some "ME" time with friends will not only provide emotional and social support, it will make you a more patient and loving caregiver.

Meditation

Try simple meditation. Meditation is a practice of spending time in quiet thought and relaxation. This practice will give you time to center and focus on you and your well-being. You can purchase a book on simple meditation or go to YouTube for easy and simple guided videos. Meditation helps to decrease stress, increase focus and revive energy. It also helps you to return to a place of peace and balance. Here is a great article on meditation. http://www.forbes.com/sites/alicegwalton/2015/02/09/7-ways-meditation-can-actually-change-the-brain/ You can also find excellent aps to help with guide mediation. Try this cool one on your iPhone:

https://itunes.apple.com/us/app/headspace-meditation-techniques/
id493145008?mt=8

Exercise

Being a long-term caregiver is like being an athlete. Treat your body well and be aware of proper body mechanics. Bend at the knees. Engage your stomach muscles before lifting, etc. With your doctor's approval, stay fit with light cardio and simple free-weight training two days a week. Those who visited Kevin and me during our ALS journey knew that several times a week I was hitting the speed bag in the garage. It relieved stress, raised endorphin levels and cleared my head. Consider recruiting a workout buddy; he or she will motivate you to make the time.

Setting Boundaries

While it is important to express your appreciation and make sure that volunteers feel welcome, you will also want to uphold a certain level of privacy in your home. The persistent flow of traffic in and out of your home can feel stressful at times if you are not a social butterfly. Carve out time each day or week to spend alone with your family. This may also mean that you need to feel comfortable saying "no." Most people are mindful of the sensitivity of the situation and will not be offended if you politely decline help or. It is acceptable to establish guidelines and then share them with your village respectfully. Consider blocking family time into your "Share the Care" weekly schedule.

Good To KNOW: Caregiving Resources are available for YOU. There are several caregiving groups on Facebook, which we have included in our Resources. If you do not like FB and would rather meet face-to-face, you could SKYPE other CALS (Caregiver of someone with ALS) or attend a support group. The ALS Association has support groups associated with various chapters. For more information, go to: www.alsa.org, go to Home page, click on In Your Community, then click on side link, Support Groups to Find a Support Group and then enter your state for a support group near you.

Personal Narrative
Of One Male Caregiver

By Warren Benton Ames

My wife Jodi asked me to share my perspective of being an ALS caregiver, specifically as a male caregiver. That apparently places me in a minority, but by no means exclusive territory. Certainly not a role I chose, and one for which I was woefully unqualified.

My family background is such that we were taught to be self-sufficient, not to rely on others for anything you could (possibly) do yourself, and most importantly don't expect too much sympathy if you managed to get hurt or get sick. We grew up in rural farming country and were very much schooled by the Depression-Era mentality. Fortunately, we never got very sick, and rarely injured ourselves badly. There were seven in our family and we were all expected to subscribe to a 'Fall Behind, Get Left Behind" philosophy. It had, and has its merits as well as drawbacks; not good, not bad. How could I have learned to be a caregiver with little or no experience?

Like most of you, I suspect, I was completely ignorant about ALS. Eventually I found out it was also known as 'Lou Gehrig's Disease'; the sum of my knowledge on that was a picture in my mind of a very healthy, very handsome Gary Cooper declaring to be 'the luckiest man in the world.' How bad could it be? I didn't even know it was a fatal disease until my wife and I came home the day she was 'officially' diagnosed and burst out crying asking, "Who is going to take care of my kids?" Just as much to the point, who was going to take care of her?!

Without a doubt, my hardest lesson was that we couldn't do this by ourselves. My job was a 75-minute commute, one way. Our two children were seven and nine at the time. How or why I thought I could manage this without too much help is absurd. The first step is to get rid of your pride. Carry that with you and the whole family will suffer. Once we began reaching out, I found we had a miraculous number of friends that I had never met. There will be people, amazing people, who will get enormous happiness from just being able to help. There is always a need for some-thing, likely something you never even considered, and you likely will need it right NOW. Miracles are rare, and there will be not be a shortage of things you need or want that you'll learn to live without. Be gracious to anyone offering help, be courageous enough to decline 'help' you cannot use if is counter-productive. Keep them close, even after your life with ALS has come and gone.

Growing up, our family had the motto "No blood, no sympathy." We laughed about it then and still do, but the feeling behind it was genuine. Sympathy, I think is a bit overrated; empathy, on the other hand needs to be tattooed on your brain. Learn to feel what your patient is feeling; learn to do your best to deal with every one of their feelings trivial or otherwise. It has been fifteen years since my wife passed, but I can remember how proud I was at the time for something she told me: we had a wheelchair ramp constructed for the house and countless people wheeled her up the ramp countless times. I happened to notice how she winced as the front wheels of the chair tapped the end of the ramp, so I of course I paused each time at the end of the ramp, lifted the front wheels over the bump, and went on. She commented that I was the only one who knew to do that for her. So trivial in the overall picture of what we had to deal with but it was (and still is for me) one of our most tender moments together.

My late wife Tina Singer Ames and I had been married almost twenty years before she was diagnosed, and I'm confident saying we had an unusually good marriage. The feelings we shared with and dealt with in those years all came back, sometimes with a vengeance. Do not allow this to destroy your relationship with each other. Guard the love you (hopefully) have with each other as the most precious thing a human being can have. It's also possible, maybe just as likely that your relationship was lacking a bit to begin with. This is the opportunity to fix that. This disease will strain every aspect of your life, and if you can both manage to face the brutal outcome loving each other, it will bring you pride and contentment every day of your remaining life. None of us can know exactly what someone else is feeling or thinking without having been in their situation. Even then, it would be just a guess. The major issues will cry out loud enough, leaving no doubt about feelings.

Keep in mind what your loved one is facing, try to remember how they have reacted and responded to stressful times in the past, and learn how to help the situation. Use what you already know about this person, anticipate what they need and do your best to provide it. With luck, maybe your loved one will have the capacity to care about your needs as well. Don't count on it, however. If you have to, just deal with it as best you can—somewhere else. Your time to be needy and comforted will come but now is not that time. Again, seek out the help you need but never use it as a weapon. Nobody wants to hear how the frequent trips to clinic interfere with your golf handicap. If nothing else, use this experience to learn what is or is not important in life.

My wife died less than ten months after being diagnosed. "Three to five years" was the estimate on life remaining, two if you are unlucky. To say I am sorry that I wasted even five minutes of that time waiting for 'the right time' to tell how much she meant to me would be an understatement of epic proportions. We were lucky to have a solid, loving marriage and I'll always regret having misspent any moment of our time together. Thinking we had some time, I never got around to telling her how much some things meant to me, and how sorry I was that I made her feel some things were so important to me. This is a proving ground for your character. You won't be perfect with every decision, there will be times you drop the ball. Dust yourself off, learn from it, and whatever it takes, make your loved one proud of you.

Warren Benton Ames

All-around great guy and husband of author/editor Jodi O'Donnell-Ames. 'Car guy' from day one. Currently, he's working 9:00-5:00 doing research work for ExxonMobil Corp. A Hope Loves Company® founding board member, Benton works to fight back against the disease that claimed his late wife Tina Singer Ames by providing the much needed help that wasn't there when his own children needed it. Camp HLC® is Warren's favorite activity because it combines his love for camping and his determination to make a difference.

CHAPTER 13

Getting Help from Your State

By Latoya Weaver, PSC

Medicare and Benefits

While there are government assistance programs available for people living with ALS, know that in order to receive help, PALS and their families must do their homework. Getting help from your insurance company and state takes research, time, energy and persistence. There will be numerous phone calls made, many extended conversations and endless questions and paperwork. The experience can be daunting and exhausting for someone in perfect health!

Benefits

Medicare benefits are made available for PALS under the age of 65. For a person to get approved for disability benefits based on a diagnosis of Amyotrophic Lateral Sclerosis (ALS), medical records must include a specific ALS diagnosis. Because there is no one test that establishes the presence of ALS, the ALS diagnosis must be made following the accepted practices and clinical procedures used to diagnose ALS, and for patient records to provide evidence of diagnosis. Your PALS' neurologist should be familiar with this process, but it never hurts to research the steps yourself. If a neurologist has made a diagnosis of ALS, Social Security should approve the PALS for disability benefits. PALS should be fast-tracked due to their ALS diagnosis under the Compassionate Allowances program. For a definition and additional information about CAL, go to www.ssa.gov/compassionateallowances/. This act means that ALS cases should be decided within a couple of weeks.

According to their website,

"Compassionate Allowances allow Social Security to target the most obviously disabled individuals for allowances based on objective medical information that we can obtain quickly. Compassionate Allowances is not a separate program from the Social Security Disability Insurance or Supplemental Security Income programs. "

Medicare packages are comprised of four parts, conveniently named Part A, B, C, and D. These parts refer to Hospital Insurance, Medical Insurance, Medicare Advantage, and Prescription Drug Coverage, respectively. Your insurance provider can point you in the direction of a Medicare Case manager to help you with your Medicare questions. Case Managers are often nurses or social workers whose role is to serve as a mediator between you and your insurance company and provide community resource assistance.

Please know that it is important to **immediately** complete and submit your PALS' application to Social Security once a diagnosis is given because he or she must qualify for and receive Social Security Disability Insurance (SSDI) to be eligible for Medicare. Patients will automatically be enrolled in Medicare a month after receiving SSDI. Most families are unable to cover the associated medical costs without insurance, so be proactive in getting the services needed.

An excellent practice is to keep a journal and record the steps made to get assistance. Record the date of each visit, conversation and phone call. Ask for the person's name at each department to keep advice and information organized. PALS need strong advocates who are comfortable making phone calls and asking questions. A friend who understands healthcare and benefits and who is efficient in problem solving and tackling tasks is a bonus!

To apply for disability benefits, call the Social Security Administration at 800-772-1213. Depending on your preference, they will make an appointment for you to complete an application either via telephone or at your local SSA office. You can also apply for SSD benefits online at www. ssa.gov.

Veteran Benefits

Anyone who served at least 90 days of continuous active duty in the United States Military may qualify for Veteran Administration benefits. Survivors of veterans may be eligible for benefits, including monthly compensation, regardless of when their loved one was lost to the disease.

Qualifying Veterans with ALS are entitled to receive VA disability compensation, which is a monetary benefit paid to veterans who are disabled by an injury or disease that was incurred or aggravated during active military service. ALS is considered service- related due to the higher incidence of ALS in military personnel. Disability compensation is paid monthly and varies with the degree of disability and the number of veteran's dependents. Veterans with ALS may be eligible for additional special monthly compensation.

The VA offers a full range of health care benefits, including prescriptions, medical supplies, prosthetic items, home improvement and structural alteration grants to pay the cost to make the home more accessible.

Also, there are a variety of other benefits available to veterans, spouses, and children. Some benefits are available even if the veteran with ALS has passed away, such as dependency and indemnity compensation, which is a monthly payment to eligible survivors. Other veteran and family benefits include insurance benefits for dependents, special adaptive housing grants, automobile grants, adaptive equipment, along with aide and attendance allowance to pay for care providers.

To apply for Veteran benefits, please visit www.benefits.va.gov or the Paralyzed Veterans of America—www.pva.org . The Paralyzed Veterans of America currently has 69 national service offices nationwide. By contacting one of these offices, veterans can speak with a National Service Office (NSO) to ensure they are receiving benefits to which they are entitled.

Healthcare and Equipment Costs:

PALS need health insurance and the right equipment and medical supplies to live with the challenges of ALS. It is suggested that early on, seek and make friends with a caring and reliable case manager at your health insurance company. The role of a case manager is to evaluate a patient's needs and his or her available resources. The case manager should find the best, most efficient and financially possible way of meeting a PALS' needs with the resources available.

According to the MDA website: http://www.mda.org/publications/mda-als-caregivers-guide/chapter-7/help_with_costs

*"Under federal regulations, an employer's health care plan must include arrangements for continuing an employee's coverage for at least some period of time after the employee leaves the job for reasons including disability. (COBRA.) The employer also may maintain short-term and long-term disability plans for employees. Check with the company's human resources department. Private and government insurance plans cover a great deal of the medical expenses associated with ALS, but not everything. Become familiar with which policies cover what, and be prepared to **appeal denials** of coverage. "*

The key is to do your research and know PALS' rights and be proactive in obtaining the equipment and help necessary for your PALS who deserves to LIVE with ALS.

Personal Narrative

By Donna Dourney York, founder of Hark, Inc.

My dad, Charlie "Hark" Dourney was diagnosed with Bulbar ALS 18 months after taking him to numerous doctors to determine why he was slurring his words and felt like he had too much saliva in his mouth. Bulbar onset affects swallowing, speaking and breathing before it starts to affect the limbs. My dad lost his ability to speak 6 months after diagnosis, he communicated with a dry erase board. Swallowing slowly deteriorated until the point where he had to choose whether or not to get a feeding tube. We sat down with him as a family to discuss his decision, he knew the disease would progress faster without one but he didn't want one. It was hard for us but we had to respect his decision, as it was his to make. The hardest part about this for my dad was that he had to let his 7 children, whom he had taken care of for more than half of his life, now take care of him. He was also an amazing athlete, slowly losing the ability to use his muscles as he had for so long, was terrifying. He was the strongest man I've ever known, he fought every day as his muscles slowly started to shut down, but he was no match for ALS and passed away 18 months after diagnosis, November 2, 2009.

I started Hark, Inc. in 2011 in his memory. My family and I lived close enough to my dad to help with his care. He was a veteran so he received benefits from the VA. He worked hard his whole life so he had a retirement pension as well as Medicare and AARP insurance so we really had all of the resources we needed to take care of him and keep him at home until he passed away. It was heartbreaking to watch, the strongest man in the world in my eyes, slowly waste away from this debilitating disease. But my family is very close and we did what we always do, we came to together and took care of each other and him.

Not long after my dad passed away, my friend's husband was diagnosed with ALS. They had no health insurance because he was unable to work. As a result, they struggled financially. Their house was in foreclosure and she eventually had to quit her job to stay home and take care of him. He passed away not long after diagnosis and she was devastated financially.

I thought often of them as I considered starting an ALS organization and what the needs were of ALS families that were not being met by other organizations. I decided to create Hark to provide financial support to patients and their families. I thought often of how I would have ever been able to take care of my dad and keep him home if it was just me and he did not have the financial security that he did. It would have been overwhelming to say the least.

When I started Hark, my first thought was, how do I raise funding for a disease most people know nothing about? The opportunity came up to film a documentary and so I jumped in with both feet. It took us 2 years to raise the funds and film Hope on the Horizon: An Expedition for ALS. Our NY premiere was held at NBC Universal in NYC and our NJ premiere was held at the Shakespeare Theater at Drew University. The film has been screened at several film festivals, but more importantly, we use it to raise funding to support local ALS families as well as our funding for Hark, Inc. We share the film at every opportunity and our goal is to change the way the world views ALS and inspire others to get involved and help.

We have been able to provide support for several ALS families through our documentary by hosting screenings in areas across the country where the entire community comes out to support the family. This enables us to educate the community members on what the family is facing as the disease progresses and creates a network of support beyond a one-time event. All proceeds from the events are given to the family.

Hark established a scholarship in memory of Elaine Stewart Tyrell, a police officer who lost her battle with ALS one year after diagnosis and a grant in memory of Captain Stanford H. Shaw III, to be given to a military family battling ALS. Captain Shaw was killed in a military training exercise; he was a great friend and supporter of Hark, Inc.

We've been able to provide assistance to several families that were struggling financially to pay their bills, others that wished to visit their families for a special occasion and didn't have the money to go, and help for those that could not pay for what they needed to continue their battle with ALS. We are able to quickly respond to the needs of people with ALS while incorporating the beneficiary's vision of what will improve his or her quality of life.

We provided scholarships for children to attend Camp HLC and will be hosting an additional camp with Hope Loves Company for a free camp for children and grandchildren of ALS patients.

Donna Dourney York

Donna has a BS in Health, PE & Recreation form Seton Hall University, a MS in Management from the College of St. Elizabeth and a Certification in Non-Profit

Management from Rutgers University. Donna is one of 7 kids in a big Irish family.

When her dad was diagnosed with ALS the family came together, as it always did, and took care of him at home until his passing 18 months after diagnosis. Donna often thought, "What if I was an only child, what if I had to do that alone, it would be overwhelming!" Those thoughts inspired her to start Hark, Inc., a non-profit dedicated to raising awareness of ALS and ensuring that no one has to make the journey through ALS alone. The Hark family will become their family. Hark, Inc. has helped many families to alleviate the financial hardships that come with battling ALS. Donna lives in Hillsborough with her husband Ken and between them they have 6 grown children and 4 grandchildren.

Resources

ALS Books

For Children:

What Did You Learn Today? by Tina Singer Ames—Written by a person with ALS, this book gently explains ALS to younger children by following the progression of the disease as it affects an elementary school teacher, Mrs. Meyer.

The Stars that Shine by Jodi O'Donnell-Ames—Sarah has a problem. Every year she and her father march in the Fourth of July Parade. This year is different. Sarah's daddy is sick and can no longer walk. To make matters worse, he relies on a wheelchair, an UGLY wheelchair. Sarah has to decide whether she will listen to her pride and break a father-daughter tradition or listen to her heart and embrace a new one.

Momma Zooms by Jane Cowen-Fletcher—A small boy, with the aid of his energetic mother, her wheelchair "zooming machine," and a bit of imagination, pretends that he is on a train, a spaceship, and more.

My Grampy Can't Walk by Vanita Oelschlager—Grampy has multiple sclerosis and uses a wheelchair, but that doesn't keep him from doing some pretty spectacular things with his grandchildren in this inspiring and enlightening story.

Caitlin's Wish by Victoria Taylor (father is sick)—Author Victoria Taylor began writing as a way of helping her young daughter come to terms with her father's rare brain condition, Caitlin's Wish was published in 2010 in the hope of helping other children as well. It soon became apparent that people of all ages were reading the book; whole families were using it to open the discussions into their personal situations.

Tear Soup: A Recipe for Healing After Loss by Pat Schwiebert

Rachel and the Upside Down Heart by Eileen Douglas—*Rachel and the Upside Down Heart* is a magnificent and compelling true story that will open the hearts and minds of both children and parents. When Rachel is four years old, her daddy dies, and Rachel's life changes forever. She and her mommy travel from their house in Kentucky to the busy streets of New York City. At first Rachel feels so sad that it's as if her heart is upside down, But after a while Rachel discovers happiness again without forgetting her daddy.

Teens/ Adults:

Tuesdays with Morrie by Mitch Albom—Former student and current writer Mitch Albom journals his Tuesdays with his friend Morrie Schwartz, who lives with ALS.

Just to Make You Smile by Sarah Caldwell—With a special foreword by former pro-football player Steve Gleason, Just To Make You Smile is the rare, honest, compassionate and bold account of a young adult's process of watching a parent get ill and die, and the inspiration she hopes to impart by sharing her grieving process, deep inner growth, and healing.

Until I Say Goodbye by Susan Spencer-Wendel—Susan Spencer-Wendel's Until I Say Good-Bye: My Year of Living with Joy is a moving and inspirational memoir by a woman who makes the most of her final days after discovering she has amyotrophic lateral sclerosis (ALS).

Last Flight Out: Living, Loving and Leaving by Phyllis A. Langton—Memoir and a passionate love story, one that deepens as Phyllis and her husband George Thomas live their way into the experience of ALS, its unremitting losses and its surprising gifts, with dignity, keen humor, a fighter pilot's courage and a nurse's unsentimental pragmatism.

Learning to Fall by Philip Simmons—Philip Simmons was just thirty-five years old in 1993 when he learned that he had ALS, or Lou Gehrig's disease and was told that he had less than five years to live. As a young husband and father, and at the start of a promising literary career, he suddenly had to learn the art of dying. Nine years later, he has succeeded, against the odds, in learning the art of living.

Traveling to Infinity: The True Story Behind the Theory of Everything by Jane Hawking—In this compelling memoir, Stephen Hawking's first wife, Jane Hawking, relates the inside story of their extraordinary marriage. As Stephen's academic renown soared, his body was collapsing under the assaults of a motor neuron disease. Jane's candid account of trying to balance his 24-hour care with the needs of their growing family reveals the inner strength of the author, while the self-evident character and achievements of her husband make for an incredible tale presented with unflinching honesty.

Share The Care, How To Organize a Group to Care for Someone Who Is Seriously Ill by Sheila Warnock & the late Cappy Capossela. Read more information about STC, see Chapter 11.

Support for Children

Websites:

Good Grief—NJ: Good Grief provides FREE support to children, teens, and young adults after the death of a mom, dad, brother, or sister. Their programs help participants develop the coping skills they need now and for the future.
www.good-grief.org/

American Association of Caregiving Youth: Caregiving Youth are children and adolescents who are 18 years of age or younger and who provide significant or substantial assistance, often on a regular basis, to relatives or household members who need help because of physical or mental illness, disability, frailty associated with aging, substance misuse, or other condition. www.aacy.org

Hope Loves Company®: a non-profit whose mission is to provide educational and emotional support to the children and grandchildren of PALS. (see the *Founding Hope Loves Company* chapter in this book). www.hopelovescompany.com

ALS Organizations

The ALS Hope Foundation—(see the *ALS Hope Foundation* chapter in this book). www.alshopefoundation.org

The ALS Association—Established in 1985, The ALS Association is the only national non-profit organization fighting Lou Gehrig's Disease on every front. www.alsa.org

Hark, Inc.—Hark, Inc. is an active ALS charity organization that was founded by Donna Dourney York in memory of her father, Charles W. Dourney, a lifelong athlete, coach, and father of seven, who courageously battled ALS until his death in November 2009, and who was affectionately known as "Hark" by his wife Ann. www.hark-als.org

Les Turner ALS Foundation—Since 1977, the Les Turner ALS Foundation has been Chicagoland's leader in patient services, research, and education for Amyotrophic Lateral Sclerosis (ALS) and other motor neuron diseases (MND) www.lesturnerals.org

Kevin Turner Foundation—The Kevin Turner Foundation (KTF) was created to bring attention to ALS and sports-related traumatic brain injuries. www.kevinturnerfoundation.org

Team Gleason—Steve and his friends and family started Team Gleason to generate public awareness for ALS, raise funding to empower those with ALS to live a rewarding life, and ultimately find a cure. www.teamgleason.org

ALS Therapy Development Institute—The ALS Therapy Development Institute and its scientists actively discover and develop treatments for ALS.

We are the world's first and largest nonprofit biotech focused 100 % on ALS research. Led by people living with ALS and their families, we understand the urgent need to slow and stop this disease. ww.alstdi.org/

Stay Tough. Fight Hard—staytough. fightHARD. Inc. is a grassroots non-profit organization. The origin of staytough. fightHARD was a fundraiser to benefit Timothy M. O'Neill Jr. The benefit was organized by Timothy's fellow classmates; Nick Mauritz, Becky Fisher, Ellen Kurkowski, and Jon Hemmert. Upon the successful completion of the benefit, it was decided to expand stay tough. fightHARD. into a non-profit organization for education, fundraising and medical assistance.

MDA—The Muscular Dystrophy Association is the world's leading nonprofit health agency dedicated to finding treatments and cures for muscular dystrophy, amyotrophic lateral sclerosis (ALS) and other neuromuscular diseases. www.mda.org

KICK ALS! Founded by Tom Fraehmke, an organization that brings Soccer fans, players, referees and coaches together to raise funds and help find a cure for ALS. www.kickals.org

Christopher and Dana Reeve Paralysis Resource Foundation—The Christopher & Dana Reeve Foundation is dedicated to curing spinal cord injury by funding innovative research, and improving the quality of life for people living with paralysis through grants, information and advocacy. http://www.christopherreeve.org

International Alliance of ALS/MND—The International Alliance of ALS/MND Associations was founded in 1992 to provide an international community for individual ALS/MND Associations from around the world. Our vision is to engage with our members, prospective members, and other organizations to share resources globally, advance awareness and support people with ALS/MND worldwide. www.alsmndalliance.org

A.L.S. Family Charitable Foundation—The A.L.S. Family Charitable Foundation was started in 2001 in hopes of creating a brighter future for those living with A.L.S. in New England and honors all of the courageous individuals and families touched by this disease. www.alsfamily.org

Brigance Brigade—The Brigance Brigade Foundation's mission is to equip, encourage, and empower people living with ALS. We strive to improve the quality of life for patients and their families by providing access to needed equipment, resource guidance and support services. www.brigancebrigade.org/

ALS Therapy Alliance—The ALS Therapy Alliance (ATA) was established in 2000 to facilitate ALS research projects and collaborations among a diverse group of scientists and clinicians at multiple institutions to cure ALS. This represents a unique collaborative enterprise that spans single laboratories and universities. www.alstherapyalliance.org/

Support for Caregivers:

These links are great for information and support:

- https://www.facebook.com/groups/alscaregivers/ (for all caregivers)
- https://www.facebook.com/groups/339792799440638/ (for all caregivers)
- https://www.facebook.com/groups/783085008445585/ (tips and support)
- https://www.facebook.com/groups/773825372686599/ (for spousal support)
- http://www.alsa.org/als-care/caregivers/caregiving-tips-and-hints.html?referrer=https://www.google.com/

Share The Care™ is a highly regarded grassroots model that provides people with the roadmap on how to pool their talents, time, and resources to assist a friend or loved one (of any age) facing a health, aging or medical crisis and importantly how to maintain their help over time. Family caregivers find support without adding to health insurance and home health care costs and avoid caregiver burnout. Share The Care™ has been used extensively in the US and other countries to support people with ALS, (MND) their caregivers and families. And for people who live alone with no family (nearby) having a "created family" is critical when illness strikes. www.sharethecare.org

Well Spouse Association—Providing peer support and education about the special challenges and unique issues facing "well" spouses every day. www.wellspouse.org

Grief Support

griefspeaks.com

griefshare.org

hospicenet.org

nationalwidowers.org

hellogrief.org

www.nationalallianceforgrievingchildren.org/

Carole Brody Fleet, who lost her husband to ALS, has written several helpful resources for widows. About her book *Widows Wear Stilettos: A Practical and Emotional Guide for the Young Widow*—"Widowhood is a frightening prospect for any woman, but becoming a widow in one's forties, thirties, or twenties can be terrifying. *Widows Wear Stilettos* deals sensitively with the many problems and questions facing the young widow: depression and grief, helping children cope, facing in-laws, and returning to work. The author also addresses practical concerns including financial considerations and personal issues such as health, self-awareness, diet, and exercise. This reassuring book shows how a life that feels at an end can begin anew." www.amazon.com/Carole-Brody-Fleet/e/B002IU5KPK

ALS Clinics in the US:

ALS Association approved Clinics: http://www.alsa.org/community/als-clinics/

MDA approved Clinics: https://www.mda.org/services/your-mda-clinic

ALS Residences in the US:

ALS Residence Initiative—ALSRI seeks to inspire mission-driven non-profit nursing homes to build homes for people with ALS (PALS) that are residential and provide 24 hour skilled care that is as compassionate and consistent as your own family within an environment that is fully automated and prepared to provide vent support to allow PALS and people who are similarly disabled to live with their disability instead of die of it. http://www.alsri.org

Specialized Residence for PALS—The Steve Saling ALS Residence in Chelsea, MA (Boston) www.alsri.org/saling-residence.html

The Team Gleason House for Innovative Living
http://www.teamgleason.org/team-gleason-house

ALS Forums and Chats

Open support community for people affected by ALS/MND. ALS Forums—The ALS support forum is an all-volunteer driven resource provided free of charge to help anyone directly or indirectly affected by ALS and MND (also known as Lou Gehrig's disease). www.alsforums.com/

International Alliance of ALS/MND Associations—The International Alliance of ALS/MND Associations was founded in 1992 to provide an international community for individual ALS associations from around the world. Its vision is to engage with their members and other organizations, to share resources globally, advance awareness and support PALS worldwide. Their directory includes contact information for associations in more than 30 countries. www.alsmndalliance.org/

PatientsLikeMe—PatientsLikeMe is a patient-powered research network that aims to improve lives and a real-time research platform that aims to advance medicine. www.patientslikeme.com

Assistive Technology Resources

ALS Assistive Technology Blog—Alisa Brownlee, ATP's blog offers recent articles and web information on ALS assistive technology, including augmentative alternative communication (AAC), computer access, and other electronic devices that can impact and improve quality of life for people with ALS. See also: @alsassistivetec on Twitter.
http://alsassistivetechnology.blogspot.com/

AT Educational Webinar by Sara M Feldman, PT, DPT, ATP:
http://www.alsconsortium.org/educational_webinars.php

Amy and pALS Amy Roman, MS, CCC-SLP is an Augmentative Communication Specialist at Forbes Norris ALS Research and Treatment Center. Her blog Amy and pALS offers ALS speech and communication solutions, plus tips from various ALS experts. www.amyandpals.com

Equipment exchange:
https://www.facebook.com/groups/ALSEquipmentExchange/

Clinical Trials and Research updates:

The Northeast ALS Consortium (NEALS) Clinical Trials Database—
NEALS' mission is to rapidly translate scientific advances into clinical research and new treatments for people with Amyotrophic Lateral Sclerosis (ALS) and motor neuron disease (MND).

ALS Association Research Program—The ALS Association has committed $99 million to find effective treatments and a cure for Lou Gehrig's Disease.

ALS Therapy Development Institute—Webinars each month, ALS TDI brings together researchers from their lab and others for a conversation about an important topic to patients today. These can be on a specific trial, an emerging technology, or a broad theory gaining notoriety in the effort to combat ALS.

ALS Untangled—ALS Untangled helps patients with amyotrophic lateral sclerosis (ALS) to review alternative and off-label ALS treatments. Instructions for using ALSUntangled, as well as their published and active reviews can all be found on this website. www.alsuntangled.com

MDA/ALS Newsmagazine—This magazine features the latest in ALS research news from the Muscular Dystrophy Association.

The MND Research Blog (UK)—This blog aims to provide you with up-to-date information as well as the latest news on ALS/MND research. www.mndassociation.org/research/mnd-research-blog/

The National ALS Registry—The National Amyotrophic Lateral Sclerosis (ALS) Registry program, launched in October 2010, now includes registrants from all 50 states, according to the ATSDR. The registry collects information on PALS by using both existing data and self-registration.

Project MINE—To understand the genetic basis of ALS and to ultimately find a cure for this devastating, fatal neuromuscular disease, Project MinE aims to analyse the DNA of at least 15,000 ALS patients and 7,500 control subjects. The resulting 22,500 DNA profiles will be compared.

Movies And Documentaries

Hope on the Horizon

The 48 highest peaks in the White Mountains of New Hampshire, also known as the "4000 footers", cover over 250 miles of various terrain and over 70,000 feet of elevation. Four hikers, including the filmmaker, set out to summit all 48 in a single trip on foot, two completed the journey and reached the 48th summit in 24 days to raise awareness and funding for ALS patients and their families. www.hark-als.org/hope-on-the-horizon.html

I Am Breathing

Scottish documentary and winner of a British Academy Scotland Award for Best Director. Within a year, Neil Platt goes from being a healthy 30-something British bloke with a great sense of humour to becoming completely paralysed from the neck down, thanks to the devastating illness he has inherited—known as ALS, MND, or Lou Gehrig's Disease. I AM BREATHING reminds us what it is to be alive—a tale of fun and laughs with a smattering of upset and devastation.

Climb For Kevin

Documentary chronicling former Alabama and NFL great, Kevin Turner's struggle with ALS, and what happens when a team of people, choose to honor him by climbing the tallest mountain in Africa, Mt. Kilimanjaro. The story is told by none other than legendary, Hall of Fame Coach, Mike Ditka.

Hope For Steve

Documentary about a young couple's triumphant love story while battling the husband's devastating diagnosis of ALS is growing across the nation. www.linkedin.com/company/hope-for-steve-film

The Theory of Everything

Based on the story of Stephen Hawking, winner of the Academy Award for Best Actor, a film adapted from the memoir *Travelling to Infinity: My Life with Stephen* by Jane Wilde Hawking, which deals with her relationship with her ex-husband, theoretical physicist Stephen Hawking, his diagnosis of motor neuron disease, and his success in physics

Much So Fast

A documentary written and directed by Academy Award nominees Steven Ascher and Jeanne Jordan. This film premiered in competition at the 2006 Sundance Film Festival, and won the Audience Award at the Boston Independent Film Festival.

You're Not You

American drama starring Hilary Swank centered on a classical pianist who has been diagnosed with ALS and the brash college student who becomes her caregiver.

TransFatty Lives

A film by and about Patrick Sean O'Brien, who lives with ALS which debuted at Tribeca Film Festival 2015. www.transfattylives.com

Veteran Assistance

VA: http://www.va.gov/opa/publications/benefits_book.asp

Paralyzed Veterans of America -A veteran service organization (VSO) such as Paralyzed Veterans of America (PVA), American Legion or Disabled American Veterans (DAV) (Contact information for VSO's can be found here: http://www.pva.org

On ALS Association website:
http://www.alsa.org/assets/pdfs/advocacy/vso_contact.pdf.

ALS News Updates

http://alsn.mda.org/

http://als-advocacy.blogspot.com/

http://alsworldwide.org/whats-new

Glossary

I. ANATOMICAL DEFINITIONS

Anterior horn cell: Motor neurons in the anterior gray column of the spinal cord (the front section of the lateral ventricle of the brain), which project to skeletal muscles.

Bulbar muscles: Muscles that control speech and swallowing.

Cervical cord: The highest part of the spinal cord.

Corticospinal tract: A tract of nerve cells that carries motor commands from the brain to the spinal cord and to the target muscle or organ. Also called the motor system, it is primarily responsible for transmitting signals for voluntary and skilled movements.

Lower motor neuron (LMN): A nerve cell that extends from the spinal cord to a skeletal muscle. All voluntary movement relies on spinal lower motor neurons, which innervate skeletal muscle fibers. LMNs control movement in the legs, arms, chest, face, throat, and tongue.

Lumbar spinal cord: The lowest part of the spinal cord.

Motor neurons: Neurons that originate in the spinal cord and synapse with muscle fibers to directly or indirectly control the contraction or relaxation of muscles, which usually leads to movement.

Motor system: The division of the central nervous system that handles voluntary and involuntary movement.

Oropharynx: The part of the throat that is located at the back of the mouth.

Thoracic Cord: The middle part of the spinal cord.

Thoracic diaphragm: A sheet of internal skeletal muscle that stretches across the bottom of the thoracic cavity (which houses the heart and lungs).

Upper motor neuron (UMN): A nerve cell that originates in the motor cortex of the brain and terminates within the medulla (another part of the brain) or within the spinal cord. UMNs direct the lower motor neurons to produce movements such as walking or chewing.

II. SYMPTOMS AND DISORDERS

Aspiration: When material (often food, drink, throat secretions, or stomach contents) accidentally enters the lungs.

Aspiration pneumonia: Inflammation of the lungs and bronchial tubes, usually as a result of inhaling foreign matter.

Atrophy: A partial or complete wasting away of body tissue or an organ, usually due to cell degeneration.

Dysphagia: Difficulty chewing and swallowing.

Fasciculation: A slight, local, involuntary muscle contraction that often appears as a flicker of movement under the skin.

Multifocal conduction block: When failure of impulse transmission occurs along a nerve fiber, resulting in slowly progressive weakness, fasciculations, and cramping, without serious sensory involvement.

Spasticity: A muscle control disorder characterized by stiff muscles and an inability to control those muscles.

III. DEVICES AND PROCEDURES

Babinski sign: An important neurologic examination based on what the big toe does when the sole of the foot is stimulated. If the big toe goes up, that may indicate a problem with the central nervous system (CNS).

Coughalatar, or cough assist machine: A device that applies rapid pressure to the upper abdomen, forcing air out of the lungs.

EMG-NCV (Electromyogram and Nerve Conduction Studies): A test that measures the electrical activity of muscles using needle electrodes that are gently inserted into the muscle.

Endoscopy: A nonsurgical procedure that uses an endoscope, a flexible tube with a light and camera attached to it, to examine the digestive tract.

Invasive ventilation with a tracheostomy: The placement of a tracheotomy tube into the windpipe to deliver air directly into the lungs.

Irradiation of the parotid gland: The use of low-dose radiation therapy to reduce salivary flow.

Mechanical vest: A vest that vibrates rapidly and applies pressure to the chest, which loosens mucus and sends it to larger airways to be cleared by coughing or suctioning.

Nebulizer: A device used to administer medication in the form of a mist inhaled into the lungs.

Non-invasive positive pressure ventilation (NIPPV): The use of mechanically assisted breaths delivered through a nasal mask, facemask, or nasal plugs.

Palliative care: Specialized medical care given to patients who have serious or life-threatening diseases, from the time of diagnosis throughout the course of illness.

Percutaneous gastrostomy (PEG) tube: A tube that penetrates the patient's stomach through the abdominal wall to provide a means of feeding when oral intake is impossible.

Postural drainage: The practice of lying in certain positions to help drain fluid out of the lungs and reducing swelling and mucus buildup. Positions include sitting, lying on your back, stomach, or sides, or sitting or lying with your head flat, up, or down.

Spirometer: A device used to measure the volume of air inspired and expired by the lungs.

Vital capacity (VC): The maximum volume of air a person can expel from his or her lungs after a full inhalation.

IV. EXPLANATION OF POTENTIAL CAUSES OF ALS

Autoimmune dysfunction: Immune attacks on the nerve cells could cause increased motor neuron degeneration. People with ALS also have higher instances of inflammation in the brain.

Cytoskeletal protein defects: Cytoskeletal protein defects involve neurofilaments, which provide the tracks to transport important molecules up and down the axon (the elongated fiber of a nerve cell along which impulses are conducted from the cell body to other cells). It has been shown that in ALS patients, neurofilaments accumulate in the nerve cell body and axons.

Defective glutamate metabolism: Glutamate is a common chemical in the nervous system used by neurons to transmit signals between one another. Glutamate is essential for normal nerve cell function but is toxic in excess.

Free radical injury and oxidative stress: Free radicals are molecules with unpaired electrons. These unstable molecules can damage cellular structures within nerve cells. In ALS patients, free radicals can reach toxic levels, damaging cells through an attack process called oxidative stress.

Gene defects and RNA processing: Some instances of ALS can be attributed to a genetic mutation, or a mistake in the DNA sequence that usually causes the cell to produce too little protein, too much protein, or a defective protein. Any change in the normal protein can be harmful to the cell, and may cause disease. A mutation may also be harmful due to its effects on RNA, a molecule that serves as a messenger between the gene and protein. To make a protein, the cell uses the DNA gene to transcribe an RNA copy, which is used as the instructions to assemble the protein. RNA is processed in several different ways before it is used to make protein. Mistakes during the RNA processing phase may also lead to disease.

Mitochondrial dysfunction: Almost all of the body's cells host mitochondria, which produce its essential energy. When mitochondrial dysfunction occurs, some functions in the body don't work normally.

Programmed cell death (apoptosis): A form of cell death in which cells that are no longer needed or are a threat to the organism are destroyed by a regulated cell suicide process.

Protein clumping and aggregation: The aggregation of proteins that are misshapen due to damage from cell processes or through the inheritance of an abnormal DNA structure. These clumps may interfere with normal motor nerve cell functions, inducing cell death.

Founding
Hope Loves Company®

By Jodi O'Donnell-Ames

Hope Loves Company® is the result of raising three children who learned about ALS (or Lou Gehrig's Disease) as young children while a parent battled ALS. My late husband, Kevin Gerard O'Donnell, heroically battled ALS from 1995 until his death in 2001. He was funny, handsome, loving and brave. Our daughter Alina was almost three when Kevin was diagnosed. She did not understand why her daddy was different, and Kevin and I watched painfully as Alina noticed and adjusted to the many changes brought on by ALS. Alina was eight years old when Kevin lost his battle with ALS.

In 2001, I began working as Director of Communications for the ALS Hope Foundation in Philadelphia, PA. I began only three months after Kevin passed. I needed to work, and I needed to continue his fight, OUR fight against ALS. At that point of my life, it's all I knew!

While there I organized a Family Fun day for ALS patients and their grandchildren. My mother sent me an article about a newly published children's book, *What Did You Learn Today?* written by Tina Singer Ames, who lost her battle to ALS in 2000. I ordered 50 copies of the book to gift to those attending Family Fun Day. The books were hand delivered by the author's widower, Warren (Benton) Ames and his children, Nora, and Adam. The Ames family was devastated much like the O'Donnell family.

We shared common phrases like: We used to, When things were better, I remember when…

It was our need for hope and our common thread of loss that bound our families together. We soon became good friends and that friendship grew into love. It was beyond a love between a man and a woman—it was a love for survival and hopes for our children to be whole again.

In 2003, Benton and I married, and our three children were the bridal party!

We were a happy family full of hope for a future after experiencing so much pain, but we all had challenges to face. I had to learn how to not only help myself but my children who grieved at different times and in different ways. I wished that there were resources available to my children, but found none to guide me. I always kept that need in mind and vowed to one day, change that situation for other families in need.

Our name, **Hope Loves Company**®, came to mind immediately. It was clear to me that gathering in hope is much more powerful than wallowing in misery. In 2007, while still raising our children, I registered the name **Hope Loves Company**® and purchased a domain name. These initial acts committed me to my dream of making a difference.

It was not until 2011, when our children were finishing or starting college, that forming a non-profit became a reality. I began having a vision, a mission and the energy to put my goals into motion. Little did I realize the task that lie ahead and the enormous growth it would have. Eighty-hour work weeks for five years straight have taken Hope Loves Company® from a registered name to the ONLY organization that supports the children and grandchildren of PALS (Persons with ALS). At Camp HLC®, children from the ages of 8 to 21 have the chance to participate in a weekend of fun activities—rock wall climbing, critter exploration, high rope walking, bonfire sing a longs, candle making, and an ice cream social. Most of the children in attendance have a parent who is currently battling ALS (Amyotrophic Lateral Sclerosis) or Lou Gehrig's disease. Some have recently lost a parent to ALS. Camp HLC also offers opportunities for art therapy, peer and counselor support. Team Gleason Hark, Inc. and The Kevin Turner Foundation are Camp HLC® sponsors.

In additional to Camp HLC®, Hope Loves Company® offers one free family day per year in the tri-state area. This is a fun day at a family oriented park or business. Fun days give families a chance to enjoy themselves while meeting similar families and making new friends. Hope Loves Company® is managed by a nine-member volunteer board of directors and is a member of several organizations, including the Pennington Business & Professional Association, Mid Jersey Chamber of Commerce, and The International Alliance of ALS/MND Association. Hope Loves Company® was recently designated as the New Jersey Association of Student Councils sponsored charity for the 2015-2016 school year. Hope Loves Company® is a 501 c (3) non-profit. Our tax exempt number is 20-8418402.

We can be found via:

- WEB: www.hopelovescompany.com
- Facebook: https://www.facebook.com/HopeLovesCompany
- Twitter: https://twitter.com/HopeLovesCo
- Instagram: HOPELOVESCOMPANY

My desk is covered in quotes. They inspire me on the challenging days and when I am exhausted. I thank the author of this quote (author unknown):

I always wondered why someone didn't do something about that. Then I realized, I am someone!

Not a day goes by without remembering Kevin and Tina and the lessons they have given us. Hope Loves Company® was formed in their memories and is fuelled by their love for us.

The ALS Hope Foundation
Hope is on the Horizon

Founded in 1999 by Dr. Terry Heiman-Patterson and the late Dr. Jeffrey Deitch

What is the ALS Hope Foundation and what are its goals?

The ALS Hope Foundation is an independent foundation headquartered in Philadelphia devoted to making a difference in the lives of people living with ALS (PALS). Our mission is to (1) support ALS patients and their families by providing excellent and compassionate care across multiple healthcare disciplines with the goal of improving lives while living with the disease, (2) support basic and clinical research aimed at accelerating the cure, treatment and reversal of ALS, and (3) support education and other collaborative programs that foster progress towards offering a better quality of life for our patients, and an eventual cure.

The MDA/ALS Center of Hope—our clinic's commitment to our patients

Founded in 1984 by Dr. Patterson with the added support of the ALS Hope Foundation since 1999, the MDA/ALS Center of Hope at Drexel University College of Medicine (the "ALS Center"), offers PALS state of the art multidisciplinary patient care, opportunities to participate in clinical research, and programs designed to help patients, as well as their families and caregivers, maintain a higher quality of life. The MDA/ALS Center relies heavily on the ALS Hope Foundation for financial support to maintain its level of excellence.

According to the American Academy of Neurology, providing multidisciplinary care is an essential part of providing quality care to PALS. Studies have shown better symptom management, a longer life and a better quality of life in PALS cared for at multidisciplinary clinics like the MDA/ALS Center of Hope. During each visit patients at our center can expect to receive personalized care from each member of the team, including our neurologists, Dr. Terry Heiman Patterson and Dr. Anahita Deboo, and each of the following other health care professionals: the nurse practitioner/coordinator, physical and occupational therapists, assistive technology specialist, respiratory therapist, nutritionist, speech and swallowing therapist, mental health specialist, social worker/case management specialist as well as a clinical research coordinator. Each health care professional evaluates and addresses the patient's constantly changing needs as the disease progresses and impacts different functions of the patient. This care helps PALS maintain the best muscular and respiratory function possible and to anticipate upcoming needs.

Programs provided to patients within the MDA/ALS Center of Hope and/or supported by the ALS Hope Foundation include:

Loaner Closet: The MDA/ALS Center of Hope offers PALS equipment and supplies on loan for the period of time needed, after which the equipment is returned so that it can be re-loaned to other patients. Typical loaner items include communications devices (eye gaze computers), ipads, power wheelchairs, shower chairs, patient lifts, and any other equipment and supplies donated by ALS patients and families. The ALS Hope Foundation partners with the MDA to support the costs associated with the delivery, repair and maintenance of all equipment.

Assistive device modification and design: The ALS Hope Foundation supports the work of engineering students to modify and design assistive technology to meet the individualized needs of people living with ALS.

Home visit program: Home visits are provided to PALS and/or family members from various members of our multidisciplinary team specializing in ALS. The purpose of these visits is to enhance the continuity of care between clinic appointments and cover topics such as: home safety, computer access, augmentative communication needs, care plan management, end of life choices, emotional/educational counseling, ventilator withdrawal, the dying process and bereavement.

Education Programs: Education is one of the primary goals of the ALS Hope Foundation and is provided to people living with ALS, their family members and caregivers, other health care providers and other facilities or agencies that help provide care to PALS. The topics are wide-ranging and include education on ALS in general, questions specific to the different disciplines, and quality of life choices such as ventilators and tracheostomies, feeding tubes and other choices.

Physician home visits: End of life counseling and implementation of ventilator decisions.

Diaphragmatic Pacer: The MDA/ALS Center of Hope is the first center in the eastern region to offer the option of diaphragmatic pacer insertion and will be participating in the upcoming DPS trial. The diaphragmatic pacer holds promise for extending respiratory function to extend breathing independence and ultimately the lives of people with ALS.

The Kevin O'Donnell Independent Living Initiative: This program supports the development of assistive technology allowing a more independent lifestyle for PALS and has provided the initial financial support for two fully accessible hospital rooms that are designed to accommodate both the person living with ALS along with their caregiver when hospitalization is needed. These rooms are fully equipped with lifts, computers, and assistive technology to allow for a comfortable stay.

There is unanimous agreement in the medical community that the multidisciplinary approach to ALS patient care is the gold standard. However, insurance does not reimburse separately for many of the healthcare professionals involved in a patient's visit to the clinic. The ALS Hope Foundation subsidizes approximately 70% of clinic visit costs so as not to overburden PALS and their families with the additional cost and time necessary for complete care during a time when they can least afford it.

ALS Hope Foundation's commitment to support basic and clinical research programs:

Currently, the ALS Hope Foundation is actively funding and overseeing our Center's basic and clinical research*. The Center has completed more than 20 clinical trials and has participated in all stages of trial development from Phases 1 to 3. See the website for updated research studies. http://www. alshf.org/clinical-research/

The Foundation's commitment to collaborations

The ALS Hope Foundation leverages its investment by encouraging and supporting collaborations within Drexel University, with other Universities and between Investigators nationwide. The Foundation has supported the Center's team of researchers at the ALS Basic Research Laboratory at Drexel University College of Medicine (DUCOM). While the laboratory is funded through outside grants for some of its work, the animal colonies, and many new research initiatives are funded in large part through grants from the ALS Hope Foundation. This funding enables collaborations between the ALS Laboratory and other investigators at DUCOM, with other Universities including Thomas Jefferson University, Wadsworth VA, and the University of Pittsburgh to name a few.

The Foundation also supports organizations that bring investigators together for collaboration and information exchange, including: The Northeast ALS Consortium (NEALS) and the Philadelphia Institute of Neurodegenerative Disorders (PhIND), and The International Alliance of MND/ALS Associations.

NEALS is a national, independent, non-profit organization consisting of researchers who collaboratively conduct clinical research on ALS and other motor neuron diseases. Its mission is to rapidly translate scientific advances into new treatments for people with ALS and other motor neuron diseases. To accomplish this, NEALS functions as an academic research consortium, a contracted research organization, and a resource tool for ALS community. Dr. Heiman-Patterson, the founder and board president of the ALS Hope Foundation, has been named co-chair of NEALS.

PhIND was co-founded by Dr. Patterson together with the late Dr. Jeffrey Deitch and is supported by the ALS Hope Foundation. PhIND is an organization dedicated to attracting excellent scientists within Philadelphia and throughout Pennsylvania to a virtual community of investigators to collaborate on research with the goal of accelerating the pace and quality of research on neurodegenerative disorders including ALS. The Institute's goals are to (1) provide endowed support for researcher salaries and labs, (2) foster collaboration and interaction between and amongst scientists at different academic institutions, and (3) provide academic support services for researchers. The theory is that the efforts of one university alone or many institutions separately, will not create the dynamic and comprehensive research effort that will ultimately attract biotechnology companies to the field of neuroscience, and specifically neurodegenerative diseases. The goal of PhIND is to attract these companies, scientists, and further investments by establishing a collaborative team approach by researchers, who gather often, generate and share ideas, offer advice, work well with each other, and assist companies in their pursuit of cures for these diseases.

The International Alliance of MND/ALS Associations was founded in 1992 to provide an international community for individual ALS/MND Associations from around the world. The Alliance functions primarily as a forum for the exchange of information on all aspects of the disease, including research and management of care. Each year, the ALS Hope Foundation supports the Allied Professionals Forum hosted by the International Alliance, which has educated thousands of healthcare professionals throughout the world.

Advocacy

The ALS Hope Foundation is committed to advocating for improved care for people living with ALS along with increased research funding and collaborative approaches to research. In FYI, one of our board members, together with her husband who was a PALS at the time, was able to successfully change the Medicare law to remove the two-year waiting period for Medicare benefits for people with ALS. Also, through our Clinical Research Learning Institute, we have worked to give PALS the tools to join in advocacy for research. We continue to advocate for individuals living with ALS and their caregivers, and will look forward to a day when people living with ALS have full access to the resources they so rightfully deserve.

Dedications:

Jodi O'Donnell-Ames—This resource guide is dedicated to my village- too many to mention but love you all. Especially to Marge O'Donnell for introducing me to her son Kevin, to the Hope Loves Company® Board and the brave children of PALS for making Hope Loves Company® a reality, to Allison Heller for cheering me on and to Jack Tatar for believing in me.

The Team at the MDA/ALS Center of Hope, including authors Terry Heiman Patterson, Sara Feldman, Mary Paolone and Latoya Weaver and the ALS Hope Foundation—This book is dedicated to individuals with ALS and their families who have taught us the meaning of courage and inspire us to make a difference.

Donna Dourney York—This is dedicated to my dad, Charlie "Hark" Dourney. He always taught me to be the best person I can be, to share the gifts that God gave me, to help others at every opportunity I'm given, to make a difference in someone's life. He is the inspiration for Hark, Inc.

Author Bios:

Jodi O' Donnell-Ames

Jodi O'Donnell-Ames is a certified teacher, writer, massage therapist, member of Union Fire Co. and Rescue Squad and tireless advocate for Lou Gehrig's disease, or ALS (Amyotrophic Lateral Sclerosis). She is also the founder and president of Hope Loves Company®, a non-profit organization committed to helping the children and grandchildren of ALS patients. She lives with her husband Benton in NJ. Their three children are now young adults who make ALL of their parents (heavenly and earthly) proud. This is her second book. She published an ALS children's book, *The Stars that Shine*, in 2013.

Dr. Terry Heiman-Patterson, MD

After completing a six-year BS/MD program from Rensselaer Polytechnic Institute and Albany Medical College, Dr. Heiman-Patterson received her residency training in Neurology from Albany Medical College and was awarded a Muscular Dystrophy Association (MDA) clinical and research postdoctoral fellowship in Neuromuscular Diseases at the University of Pennsylvania. She started her medical practice at Hahnemann University in 1982 and became the first Medical Director of the MDA Clinic at Good Shepherd Rehabilitation Hospital in Allentown, PA, where she continues today as Medical Director. In 1984, she founded and was Co-Director of the MDA/ALS Center of Hope at Hahnemann University, one of the first multidisciplinary ALS clinics in the country and the standard of excellence against which ALS clinics are judged today. This was one of the first ALS clinic officially certified by a national organization (ALS Association) and remains a leader in the field. After serving as an Associate Professor of Neurology at Thomas Jefferson University from 1988-1996, she returned to Hahnemann University, which became Drexel University College of Medicine in 2002.

Dr. Heiman-Patterson has conducted over 24 clinical trials in ALS, helped to establish the standard of care in noninvasive ventilation of ALS patients, and has received several grants to study the cause of ALS in animal models of motor neuron disease. She has authored over 50 papers, abstracts, and correspondence on motor neuron diseases. She is a member of Executive Board of the Northeast ALS Consortium of ALS researchers and physicians (NEALS), and co-chairs the biorepository subcommittee. Dr. Heiman-Patterson served on the Medical Advisory Boards of the Myasthenia Gravis Foundation, the Philadelphia Chapter of the ALS Association, and the National ALS C.A.R.E. Program. In 2000, the Muscular Dystrophy Association honored Dr. Heiman-Patterson with the Lou Gehrig Memorial Award for outstanding service as a clinician and researcher on ALS. In 1999, Dr. Heiman-Patterson helped co-found the ALS Hope Foundation and currently serves as President of the Board. In 2014 she was elected Co-Chair of the Northeast ALS Consortium (NEALS) Executive.

Sara Feldman, PT, DPT, ATP

Sara Feldman, PT, DPT, ATP has been the Physical Therapist at the MDA/ALS Center of Hope since 1994. She received her Bachelors in Physical Therapy in 1987 from Temple University, her Masters in Environmental Science from the University of Pennsylvania in 1997, and her Doctorate in Physical Therapy from Drexel University in 2012. Prior to coming to Drexel, she was a Senior Physical Therapist on the Spinal Cord Injury team at Magee Rehabilitation Hospital. She came to Hahnemann Hospital to be on the acute neurotrauma and neurology teams. Sara works full-time for the MDA/ALS Center of Hope and in addition to clinical care she is involved in clinical trials and the use of assistive technology. Sara is co-chair of the NEALS Physical Therapy Committee along with Peggy Allred, PT,

DPT from Cedars-Sinai Medical Center in Los Angeles and is the Clinical Evaluator representative on the NEALS Executive Committee. In 2013, she was elected to the Board of Directors of the International Alliance of ALS/MND Associations. She looks forward to the day there is a cure for ALS!

Mary Paolone, MSRN

Mary Paolone, MSRN is the Clinical Nurse Counselor and has worked at the MDA/ALS Center of Hope since 2005. She graduated with a Bachelor of Nursing Degree from Villanova University in 1994 and has been focused in chronic pain and chronic illness for most of her career. While working with these populations, she gained a desire to assist others more deeply as they move along the spectrum of their diseases. Mary continued her education with a Master's Degree in Counseling Psychology from Chestnut Hill College, which has enabled her to remain present and supportive with her patients during difficult times. She states that her "life has been greatly enriched by her work at the MDA/ALS Center of Hope" and considers it a blessing and an honor to help in any way she's able.

Latoya Weaver, PSC

Latoya Weaver, PSC, received a certification in medical billing and coding from CHI. Prior to joining the MDA/ALS Center of Hope, she had the experience of caring for her mother, who lived with ALS for over six years. Latoya has first-hand knowledge of the challenges that patients and families go through when dealing with ALS and is willing to work as earnestly and passionately for the people she sees as she did for her own mother. She is incredibly motivated and passionate about helping others.

Cover photo (courtesy of Gwen Pfeifer) of the late and courageous father of two, Aaron Winborn, snuggling with his four year old daughter and cheerleader, Sabina.